Shine

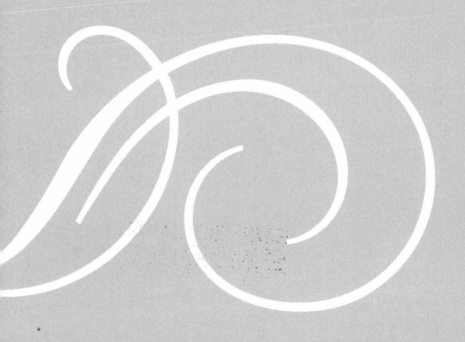

A Physical, Emotional, and
Spiritual Journey to Finding Love

Shine

Star Jones
Reynolds

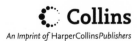

Collins
An Imprint of HarperCollinsPublishers

HarperCollins books may be purchased for educational, business, or sales
promotional use. For information please write: Special Markets Department,
HarperCollins Publishers, 10 East 53rd Street, New York, NY 10022.

FIRST EDITION

Library of Congress Cataloging-in-Publication Data has been applied for.

ISBN-13: 978-0-06-082418-1
ISBN-10: 0-06-082418-2

06   07   08   09   10   DIX/RRD   10   9   8   7   6   5   4   3   2   1

To the men in my life . . .

MY MENTORS

*Johnnie L. Cochran Jr. and Pastor A. R. Bernard, for challenging me
to be the best I could be and showing me living examples.*

MY GRANDFATHERS

Paul Faison and Clyde Bennett, for the patriarchal foundation that is our family.

MY FATHER

*James Lloyd Byard, for raising the bar so high, I had to wait for
the one who could reach it.*

MY HUSBAND

Al Scales Reynolds, for being man enough to reach that bar.

My Lord and Savior Jesus Christ . . . because he is worthy of the praise.

Contents

Preface

It should have been fine, the way my life was going should have been all I wanted, all I needed. It was such a big, full life.

So, what in the world was wrong with me?

*   *   *

I was a little girl from a tiny Southern town—Badin, North Carolina, and I was raised by a smart, loving, single-parent mother who made sure my sister and I were warm, secure, and could think for ourselves. When my mom got her college degree, we moved to the Miller Homes housing project in Trenton, New Jersey, and when I was nine, she met and later married James Byard, maybe the sweetest man on the planet. Life felt safe and I had it good. My momma Shirley named me Starlet, and early on I decided I'd shine for her, and do my best to make her proud. I still talk to her first thing in the morning, every day of my life.

I knew I was going to be a lawyer when I was eight and watching *Another World* with my grandmother Muriel. I turned to her and asked why one of the characters was always in trouble, and Mama Muriel answered, "That child just needs a good lawyer."

"What's a lawyer?" I asked.

"The ones who get people out of trouble," she answered. "You can rely on your lawyer."

"Guess I'll be a lawyer," I decided. And that was that.

After a million years in school, and after what seemed like a million dollars in loans, I fulfilled my fondest dream. I became a lawyer. I earned my BA degree at American University, got my law degree at the University of Houston, passed the New York bar, and went straight to the Brooklyn district attorney's office, ending up as senior assistant district attorney in the Homicide Bureau, where I prosecuted some pretty high-profile cases. I'd stand up in the courtroom and say, "Star Jones for the People." Were there ever before words that sang out with such clarity, strength, and courage?

"You can rely on me," I'd silently tell my grandma Muriel.

In between murder trials, I started doing volunteer commentary for Court TV. In December 1991, Court TV invited me to be the in-studio daily commentator for the William Kennedy Smith case, and I ended up with a new career as legal correspondent for television, where I covered the latest developments in media-hot cases, such as the Mike Tyson, Susan Smith, Rodney King, and O. J. Simpson trials. During this period I met the man who was to become one of my dearest mentors, the late Johnnie ("If [the glove] doesn't fit, you must acquit") Cochran.

It was fabulous and fascinating, and fame-making. Pretty heady times, sister, let me tell you.

And it would get even better as I carved out yet another career. In 1997, *The View,* a new talk show, launched. I, along with my cohosts, the legendary Barbara Walters, Joy Behar, Meredith Vieira, and Elisabeth Hasselbeck, have the time of our lives as we rap on the law, self-esteem, race, family, education, husbands, and lovers—whatever is in the news and whatever interests at least one of us. My particular job is to unmuddy muddy legal and social waters—I hate muddy waters. *The View* has received numerous awards, including the 2003 Daytime Emmy Award for Outstanding Talk Show.

So, there I was on March 24, 2003—rich (well, comfortable, not like I was

Mr. B. Gates), sort of famous, with more clothes than most boutiques, a guaranteed table in the best restaurants in town, but strangely, not very satisfied and even a little sad.

It was my birthday—I was turning forty-one. Now, I *love* my birthday so much. I'll put on a tiara, dress up, and throw the biggest bashes anyone has ever seen. So, this year, several of my closest girlfriends and I went to Jamaica for the week. The year before, on my fortieth birthday, I'd taken forty of my pals on an over-the-top, decadent, extravagant weekend, but this year I didn't seem to have the same energy. My weight, for the first time in my life, was weighing heavy on me. I'd always loved my round body, and my dress size didn't mean a thing to me because my momma and daddy always told me I was the most appealing, fine-looking woman ever born. I was proud of my breasts, my butt, my great legs, and I had more dates and more relationships than I could handle. I could always find pretty clothes in Lane Bryant even though my size went from 16 to 18, from 20 to 22. What was the big deal?

But now, for the first time in my life, I felt unhealthy. I'd gained fifty pounds in the last year and found myself unable to walk from the front of the resort to the back because it was actually painful on my knees. My overall health was getting pretty iffy, and I knew I would soon have to start making some physical changes in my life. The day I can't hang out with my best girls on the beach as much as I want to—and I couldn't on that birthday—is a bad day for me. One of my dearest friends in the world, Janet Rollé, was on that trip, and with nothing but love in her heart, she sat me down and asked the question I know a lot of my friends wanted to ask—but were too afraid.

"What's going on with you?" said Janet. "You aren't moving as well as you used to, your breathing is labored, you don't even sound healthy." And then she asked me what only a good friend could: "What are you going to do about your weight?"

When such a friend confronts you, you have to take stock. You have to stop pretending everything is fine. Then I spoke to my "godmother," Barbara Graves, who shared her private battle with weight and health. She told me to sit down, stop talking, and start listening to my body before it was too late.

So, I started listening and I started thinking. I thought about how difficult it was in church when I wanted to stand, clap, and sing out for God, but because my knees hurt, I had to remain seated. I thought about the mail I received from viewers—some mean, sure, but most so concerned because they could literally hear me breathing hard when I spoke on *The View*. I thought about how blessed I was to be able to afford to go to Paris for holiday, and yet, when I looked back on the summer before, when I'd gone to Paris, I remembered that I didn't enjoy it as much as I usually did. I couldn't walk from the plane to the terminal without getting winded, having an anxiety attack, and needing my inhalers. I didn't even feel like shopping—and that was serious. Girl, I looove shopping.

These were bad star signs.

Other things were not terrific, as well. Those relationships I just mentioned. They were wrong, just wrong. Wrong with how I wanted the relationships to end up, wrong with my own behavior: I was not true to myself—you know how you end up saying you like cats when you don't? That's stupid and that's what I found myself doing. Each time, I was trying to become someone I wasn't so I could maintain a relationship with a guy who wasn't even right for me. I wanted an extraordinary man who could and would give me the level of love and commitment I was willing to give. I know people don't love in the same way, but for me, people have to love with the same energy, the same intensity; if I'm passionate for you, you should be passionate for me. I wasn't getting back what I was giving out—it was that simple. I sure didn't need a man, but something told me that I was losing out on being a soul mate, a helpmate. I believe that is what God intended me to be.

The poet Adrienne Rich once called it "that seventh sense of what's missing against what's supplied." Much was supplied to me, but my own intuition, in which I firmly believe, told me the man of my dreams was missing. I wanted an enduring love, one that included lust, laughter, best-friendship—the deepest intimacy. I wanted a man I couldn't stop touching, one who exploded with romantic gestures. I wanted a man who would be zany over me, one who'd drive me loony with joy. I wanted a guy with whom I could find peace and safe harbor, and a little mystery wouldn't hurt, either.

I already knew what he looked like—or what I hoped he'd look like: tall, smart, passionate, handsome but not stuck-up, and careful about his appearance because I do admire a sense of style. He should be risk-taking and fun. He should have a strong relationship with his family. He should have his own thoughts and career so he won't be threatened by Star Jones Inc. He should be a spiritual person. I need to be able to trust him, totally. If you want to tell me a secret, don't ever say, "but don't tell your husband," because I will.

He should have a sweet heart.

Yeah right, Starlet. Did such a guy exist? (Oh yes, *yes*, YES!!!!!!!)

Speaking of spiritual, I wasn't doing so great in that department, either. I'm a believer in the goodness and rightness of God; I talk openly about my Christian beliefs, and I have a powerful relationship with him. Each person on this earth has to find a personal way to faith and religion—or to reject it. I respect and cherish—I'd always fight for—each one's right to believe differently. But my way is to love Christ. Most of my happiest moments find their way back to church, and it is to God whom I turn when I seek my deepest heart's joy or when I need help.

One day, near my forty-first birthday, in the makeup room at *The View*, I'd gotten called on my service to God. I was sounding off on some issue, and I made a statement about being a Christian. The next day, my friend Elena, who worked with me as my makeup artist for years, confronted me. She did it with a little trepidation—after all, I was for all practical purposes her boss—but she said, "Star, I have to share this with you. If you're going to step out for God, you have to be consistent. You have to put your life in a place where he'd be proud of the direction in which you're going."

And then, she proceeded to give me a few specifics where she thought I was failing God, one of which was the language I used. Listen—I was taught by the cops in Brooklyn, and curse words were simply normal conversation. Elena thought it wasn't consistent with my professed path of spirituality. She also told me I was being a little bit snippy with people lately. She said my attitude and interaction with others was off-putting and "un-Christ-like." And, she asked, had I noticed that I had a short fuse and was jumping way too fast to get angry with others?

I know it was hard for her to say all this because I'm not the easiest person to put in check.

I listened to her. Why? She came from a pure and honest place. I can always tell that about people.

So, there I was on my birthday, feeling far worse than I'd felt the year before, and slowly coming to realize that I'd started *not* to be the girl I wanted to be. The girl I didn't want to be was resting on her laurels. That girl thought she'd accomplished all she needed to do. She thought she was finished growing.

And she hadn't, she was nowhere near finished.

Maybe God was trying to tell me something, but I wasn't listening. Then, it all became clear.

Right after my forty-first birthday, I had a long-distance phone conversation with my best friend, Vanessa Bell Calloway, a Hollywood actress. I'd had all these successes, fans, fame, two houses, but I was still alone—not really lonely, but definitely alone. Vanessa and I were schmoozing about the Jack Nicholson movie *As Good as It Gets,* and one line in the film goes something like, "If this is as good as your life is going to get, is it good enough?" Remember that line? Vanessa said yes, she had the most wonderful family and a lovely career, and even if she never got to be the Halle Berry/Nicole Kidman/Gwyneth Paltrow type of superstar, her life was pretty spectacular and already good enough. Then, she asked me the pivotal question that would really change my life.

"If this is as good as it gets, Star, is it good enough for you?"

No. I had to say no. I didn't want to be just the girl with the cash or just the girl with the successful career. I wanted to shine inwardly as well as outwardly.

Something was clearly missing. I'm not a weepy Wanda type so I didn't cry, but I felt like it. And looking at myself clearly for the first time in my entire life, I didn't like what I saw.

I'd become complacent. I'd started resting on my laurels. Hadn't I become a hot-shot lawyer, then a television star? Wasn't that enough?

No. I'd stopped working on being the best I could be. I was awfully satisfied with Star Jones, and I couldn't afford that. We should always be shedding skin and rejuvenating. I'd stopped, I was standing still. I'd gotten lazy.

Also, I was disconnected. My expectations for what I was going to achieve had fallen, and that was the trouble, right there: I didn't have high enough expectations.

So, I went into prayer.

"God, help me to go in the direction I need to go," I prayed. "I've always come to you every time I wanted to do something careerwise. Now I need to do something personal. I give it up to you. I ask for your direction and your help."

He helped. He always did. Focus in, I heard. Assess yourself. Change your life.

Sure enough, once I recommitted myself spiritually, what I had to do physically and emotionally became clear. Like tennis balls coming at me as fast as Serena and Venus Williams could serve them, the insights came *fast*. And that's how I started to get ready to be the best I could be and, ultimately, get ready for the man who would blow me away. I had to grow, focus in, and reconstitute the three biggest areas in my life, not just to be Mrs. Someone but to be the truly fabulous Star Jones.

It took almost two years, but if you've been reading the newspapers, baby, you know it worked magnificently—in all departments. It wasn't luck, although luck always figures into life. Mostly, it took work. It always takes work.

This is what I believe: women can be many things. At different times in my life, I've been a stubborn, big-mouth kid, a daughter, a good friend, a tough lawyer, a television star—and finally now, a wife. Although I got married in my forties, I've been preparing for the wife part, preparing for Al Scales Reynolds, for a much longer time. I know that many women, by choice or fate, never marry, and that's just fine with them. For me, though, being married to someone who would complete me was a goal.

Through the last few years, I understood this: whether or not I was lucky enough to meet my soul mate, I still had to do the preparation work on *me* to make myself the best I could be. If I lucked out (and I did), my marriage would be stronger and dearer because I had so much more to offer my partner and our life together. If I never married, I would be stronger and happier alone because I'd prepared myself to be terrific. Win-win situation.

Thus, this book: I want to share my game plan with you. It isn't grim and it isn't too hard, and it's always fun and inspiring. I don't pretend to be an expert on what works for everyone, but I'm sure an expert on what doesn't work, because I've been there, done that, wrote a book, saw it on *Oprah,* and bought a T-shirt. Along with a lot of right things I did for my career, I've done everything you can possibly do wrong in certain other areas of my life. I was a complete dingbat, focusing just on work, and I didn't have an overview of who I was, where I was, and how to take better care of my physical, emotional, and spiritual needs.

But now I know what's absolute.

Absolutes

Over the course of my relationship with my spiritual advisers, Pastors A. R. Bernard and Kirbyjon Caldwell; and my "life" advisers, my grandmothers, Pauline Bennett and Muriel Faison, and my mother, Shirley Byard, they have passed on so many "words of wisdom" that I started to collect them, adapt them, and adopt them into my life. I have heard these words in some form or fashion countless times, both in a religious context and just in general conversation. What I have discovered is what my advisers figured out a long time ago: whether based in religion or not, there are some things that are just absolutes. Just true, sisters. Throughout the book, I plan to share some of those absolutes with you. Don't thank me, thank my advisers—especially Pastor Bernard. That man is no joke.

So, come along on my ride for your own transformation! I promise you it won't be boring. And if you do the work, if you prepare yourself physically, emotionally, and spiritually, you will win.

I swear it.

Part One

Be All You Can Be, Physically

Chapter 1

A Look at My (and Your) Physical Lifestyle

I decided to begin getting ready physically.

Listen—if I didn't feel or look well physically, nothing would work and I would have a snowball's chance in hell of finding my perfect mate. Physical well-being depended very much on my general lifestyle—my health, my energy level, my weight, the way I presented my physical self to the world. Even the clothes I wore, the friends and lovers I chose, the way I made decisions and dealt with anxiety—all were reflected in my physical self. Too often, I'd heard and even proclaimed, I really need to find myself. Well, if I didn't know who I was by forty, it was time to get on the stick. Of one thing I was sure: I was definitely not the best I could be. You know what? It came to me that until then, I didn't think I was ready to take complete responsibility for my lifestyle, which included that physical, emotional, and spiritual well-being. I was too busy vaulting over the top in my career. Some people are ready earlier—that's all there is to it—like my cohost Elisabeth Hasselbeck; at twenty-six she had the career, the husband, and the baby. She had a level of maturity based on personal life experiences that saw her through.

Not me—I couldn't do it all at once. But now I had a goal: because I wanted to find someone who would be my life mate, I knew I had to work on myself—make Star ready for him. But who was he?

Before I transformed myself physically, I needed an approximate visual image of my idea of a great future mate. So, I did something silly, but it worked. Just for fun, many years ago I started putting together a very specific, long list of what I wanted in a guy—and believe me, it was loooooong.

The Ideal Man for me!

Smart
Secure
Christian
Southern
Tall
Athletic build
Black
Funny
College educated
Professional
Financially Independent
Good relationship w/ his parents
Family oriented
Community Service oriented
Knows how to pray
A good dresser
Fine! (good Looking)

Sexy
No Criminal Background
No "Baby Mommas"
Likes Sports
Likes Travel
Democrat
Fiscally Responsible
Kind
Generous
Loving
Romantic
Likes Politics
A Leader
Ready for Marriage!
Billionaire

(a girl can dream)

Over the years, I added to the list, which ranged from height to weight, from background to intellect, from lifestyle to spirituality. One day on *The View*, I told my cohosts about the list. Naturally, they wanted to see it so they could make fun of me, but being a good sport, I brought it in and we talked about it on the show. I remember Barbara really taking me to task about the list.

"You'll never get it all, Star," she said. "No man can match up to this wish list."

I didn't back down; I knew what I wanted, and I kept my list. (As an aside, at our engagement party, I told everyone what Barbara had said, and I noted that I'd gotten everything but the billionaire part. "Not yet" was Al's classic response.)

I don't know what made me do this, but one day, in the middle of my own self-evaluation, I printed out the list on my computer in big, black letters, then stood at the bathroom mirror holding it right next to my body. And I asked myself: can I hold up against this man I want? The truthful answer? No. The way I looked and felt simply didn't match up to that guy. You can't ask for Denzel Washington or Clive Owen or Jimmy Smits if you're walking around looking all busted. You cannot.

Here's the deal: if you can't match up to the list, you either have to change the list or change yourself, one or the other. You have to live in the truth.

Absolute

Freedom comes the moment truth is revealed.

If you walk in truth, it is confrontational.

*You will not change in life until you are willing
to be confronted with the truth.*

I looked over my list and knew I had to live in the truth. I also knew I had the ability and, finally, the maturity—and yes, the honesty—to assess myself truthfully. I did just that—checked out my lifestyle—and came up short. For starters, I was too heavy, I was really heavy. Say it, Star—*obese,* I was obese. My clothes and makeup weren't as pretty and stylish as they used to be. And I sure wasn't making the best dating choices. No Prince Charming for Star. But, I reasoned, if I worked on it, maybe there would be someone else out there for me, someone even better than Prince Charming.

Better than the prince? It could happen. I had faith.

So, let me ask you. Could you make a list like mine? Could you figure out what you really need in a wonderful man—and what you could live without? If you want to do what Auntie Star did, the first step is to answer some vital questions, truthfully.

WHO IS HE?

How to find out:

Part I: Answer the questions. Respond to the following questions by checking the answer closest to the truth.

Part II: Decide each question's importance. Evaluate its importance to you based on the following:

    1—Absolutely mandatory
    2—Important
    3—Somewhat important
    4—A factor
    5—Doesn't matter at all

Question	Importance	Ranking
1. What is his education level?		
Answers	High school	1 2 3 4 5
	College	1 2 3 4 5
	Graduate school	1 2 3 4 5

Question	Importance	Ranking

2. What is his relationship with God?

Answers	Intense	1 2 3 4 5
	Moderate	1 2 3 4 5
	Nonexistent	1 2 3 4 5

3. What is his faith?

Answers	Christian	1 2 3 4 5
	Muslim	1 2 3 4 5
	Jewish	1 2 3 4 5
	Spiritual	1 2 3 4 5
	Atheist	1 2 3 4 5

4. Where is he from?

Answers	South	1 2 3 4 5
	Northeast	1 2 3 4 5
	Southwest	1 2 3 4 5
	West Coast	1 2 3 4 5

5. What is his height?

Answers	Tall	1 2 3 4 5
	Short	1 2 3 4 5
	Average	1 2 3 4 5

6. What ethnic group does he belong to?

Answers	Black	1 2 3 4 5
	White	1 2 3 4 5
	Hispanic	1 2 3 4 5
	Asian	1 2 3 4 5
	Mixed race	1 2 3 4 5

7. What is his relationship with his family?

Answers	Very good—speak all the time	1 2 3 4 5
	Good—meet on holidays	1 2 3 4 5
	Fair—talk and/or get together when necessary	1 2 3 4 5
	Nonexistent—don't know one another's phone numbers	1 2 3 4 5

continued

Question	Importance	Ranking

8. What is his body type?

Answers	Long and lean	1 2 3 4 5
	Athletic and muscular	1 2 3 4 5
	Nice and average	1 2 3 4 5
	Thick and cuddly	1 2 3 4 5
	Short and compact	1 2 3 4 5

9. What does he look like?

Answers	Gorgeous! (Denzel Washington, Clive Owen, Tom Cruise, Jimmy Smits)	1 2 3 4 5
	Handsome (Nice-looking, but not movie-star looks)	1 2 3 4 5
	Average (Your mother would approve and your children will look good)	1 2 3 4 5
	Quirky (You like him—so what if people don't get his look)	1 2 3 4 5
	Different (Well . . . it's his look)	1 2 3 4 5

10. What kind of music does he prefer?

Answers	Hip-hop and R & B	1 2 3 4 5
	Pop	1 2 3 4 5
	Rock	1 2 3 4 5
	Country	1 2 3 4 5
	Gospel	1 2 3 4 5
	Standards	1 2 3 4 5
	Classical	1 2 3 4 5

11. Does he have children?

Answers	Has children with ex-wife (-wives)	1 2 3 4 5
	Has children with ex-girlfriend(s)	1 2 3 4 5
	Has no children	1 2 3 4 5

12. Does he want children?

Answers	Yes, definitely	1 2 3 4 5
	Maybe	1 2 3 4 5
	No	1 2 3 4 5

Question	Importance	Ranking

13. What is his marital history?

Answers		
	Single, never married	1 2 3 4 5
	Divorced	1 2 3 4 5
	Separated, divorce pending	1 2 3 4 5
	Widowed	1 2 3 4 5
	His wife doesn't understand him	1 2 3 4 5

14. What would he do at a sporting event?

Answers		
	Play	1 2 3 4 5
	Watch	1 2 3 4 5
	Not be there	1 2 3 4 5

15. Where would he prefer to go on vacation?

Answers		
	Paris	1 2 3 4 5
	Bahamas	1 2 3 4 5
	Camping	1 2 3 4 5
	The living room	1 2 3 4 5

16. What is his political affiliation?

Answers		
	Democrat	1 2 3 4 5
	Republican	1 2 3 4 5
	Libertarian	1 2 3 4 5
	Independent	1 2 3 4 5

17. Smoking

Answers		
	Smokes habitually	1 2 3 4 5
	Smokes occasionally	1 2 3 4 5
	Has never smoked	1 2 3 4 5
	Smoked but quit	1 2 3 4 5

18. Drinking

Answers		
	Drinks frequently	1 2 3 4 5
	Social drinker	1 2 3 4 5
	Doesn't drink	1 2 3 4 5
	Recovering alcoholic	1 2 3 4 5

continued

Question	Importance	Ranking
19. Drug use		
Answers	No illegal drug use ever	1 2 3 4 5
	Has tried marijuana	1 2 3 4 5
	Uses marijuana regularly	1 2 3 4 5
	Has tried hard drugs	1 2 3 4 5
	Uses hard drugs regularly	1 2 3 4 5
	Recovering addict	1 2 3 4 5
20. Personal hygiene		
Answers	Wears cologne	1 2 3 4 5
	Clean and fragrance-free	1 2 3 4 5
	Sweat	1 2 3 4 5
21. On a Saturday night he'd prefer to		
Answers	Go to a nightclub and dance	1 2 3 4 5
	Go out for a romantic dinner	1 2 3 4 5
	Go to a movie and grab a burger	1 2 3 4 5
	Take in a sporting event	1 2 3 4 5
	Stay in and watch television	1 2 3 4 5
22. What is his annual income?		
Answers	$25,000–50,000	1 2 3 4 5
	$50,000–$75,000	1 2 3 4 5
	$75,000–$100,000	1 2 3 4 5
	$100,000+	1 2 3 4 5
	$1,000,000+	1 2 3 4 5
23. What does he want from the relationship?		
Answers	A casual friend	1 2 3 4 5
	A booty call	1 2 3 4 5
	A live-in relationship	1 2 3 4 5
	Marriage	1 2 3 4 5

Now rank these attributes in order of importance to you and add them to your list accordingly:

1. Kind   1 2 3 4 5
2. Generous   1 2 3 4 5
3. Affectionate   1 2 3 4 5
4. Romantic   1 2 3 4 5
5. Sexy   1 2 3 4 5
6. Funny   1 2 3 4 5
7. Smart   1 2 3 4 5
8. Happy   1 2 3 4 5
9. Stable   1 2 3 4 5
10. Adventurous   1 2 3 4 5
11. Assertive   1 2 3 4 5
12. Strong   1 2 3 4 5
13. Talkative   1 2 3 4 5

Finally, evaluate the following attributes as deal breakers (under no circumstances will you accept someone who . . .) and add them to the top of your list:

1. Has children already   1 2 3 4 5
2. Has a criminal record   1 2 3 4 5
3. Has violent tendencies   1 2 3 4 5
4. Uses vulgar or abusive language   1 2 3 4 5
5. Has poor personal hygiene   1 2 3 4 5
6. Can't fix a VCR/DVD or anything with a cord   1 2 3 4 5
7. Doesn't like animals   1 2 3 4 5
8. Doesn't believe in God   1 2 3 4 5
9. Is of a different faith   1 2 3 4 5
10. Is of a different ethnic background   1 2 3 4 5
11. Is skinny   1 2 3 4 5
12. Is overweight   1 2 3 4 5
13. Doesn't want children   1 2 3 4 5
14. Is unemployed   1 2 3 4 5
15. Lives with his mother   1 2 3 4 5
16. Is in debt   1 2 3 4 5
17. Knows nothing about sports   1 2 3 4 5

continued

18. Knows nothing about politics or current affairs	1	2	3	4	5
19. Knows nothing about art and culture	1	2	3	4	5
20. Is married	1	2	3	4	5

Now you have the list of what you want in the ideal man. No answer is right or wrong—they just reflect your feelings. Print the list out in large letters and let it sit. Come back to it, reevaluate it, and then make adjustments. When you have done this a couple of times, this is the list you will hold up to yourself, and then decide: do I match up to this list? If you do, go for it, girl. If not, well, you have two choices: change yourself or change the list.

* * *

There is this urban legend that a woman over forty has a better chance of being killed by terrorists than getting married for the first time. I don't think the statistic is accurate . . . but the point is. Society thinks that when you hit the big 4-0 you may as well hang it up because your days are numbered. I was determined to prove this wrong. I didn't plan to change my list, so I had to change myself. I wanted love in my life, but first I needed to love my life. A man, even the ideal one on that list, couldn't do it for me. That was my job.

The Art of Self-Assessment

Self-reverence, self-knowledge, self-control,
These three alone lead life to sovereign power.

ALFRED, LORD TENNYSON

I may have had a lot of work to do in that job of changing myself, but I already knew those three things Tennyson talked about. It was important, yes, to revere and celebrate yourself—who would love and honor you if you weren't proud of whom you'd become? It was equally important to be able to control yourself—

when it came to many things like overeating, overspending, and over—mouthing off. But maybe the most important trait a person could pick up in her years was self-knowledge, which included the ability to honestly assess herself so she would know where she had to change—if her happiness depended on change.

> ## Absolute
> ∽
>
> *You can't break away from a* pattern *unless you solve the* problem.

Many of us have blind spots that cause us to make the same mistakes over and over. We just can't see what we're doing wrong, and we even fall into patterns—like constantly picking the same guys who are terrified of making commitments or who spend our money without putting their hands in their own pockets.

And here's the really bad news: these patterns are set in stone unless we solve the problems within ourselves that provoke us into picking loser guys or wearing crude, flashy makeup or eating chips until we self-destruct. One of our tasks in preparing ourselves physically is to erase those blind spots so we can see ourselves clearly. First step: learn to assess yourself with honesty. It takes practice.

Unless you're in serious denial, no one's going to be as honest about yourself as you. I think we all have self-knowledge implanted in our genes, but too often, we choose to ignore the truth so we can look a little better to ourselves. Certainly, your mom may shade the truth a bit when you ask her if she thinks you're fat, because she loves you so much she doesn't want to hurt your feelings. Your friend may feel uncomfortable about telling you that no one can see your green eyes because the intense blue eye shadow trumps everything else on your face, or that the cute velvet bow in your hair belongs on a preschooler, not on a grown woman. And if you ask the new guy you just met (is he the one—is this true love?) what he thinks is your weakest point, he is not going to want to go there.

So, in order to be in control of your physical presentation—because make no mistake, that's what you're offering the world, a presentation of you—you need to be able to fairly judge what the mirror, your sense of well-being, and your instincts tell you.

Martin Luther King said something I love that I think applies here: "We cannot prevent birds from flying over our heads," said the Reverend King, "but we can keep them from making nests on top of our heads." Dr. King knew we couldn't prevent outside influences from affecting us, sometimes negatively—your skin might break out with a humongous pimple before the audition, the zipper on your jeans may tear at a very inopportune time, humidity might result in a really bad hair day, and stress may point the way to eating six slices of bacon. However, if we see ourselves clearly, if we truthfully assess the way we present to the world, we can cut our losses and do major damage control.

If you prepare for most contingencies, know where your weaknesses lie, and anticipate disaster, no bird's going to make a nest in your hair, honey. The pimple can be disguised with clever makeup, you know size 12 jeans on size 18 hips is asking for trouble even if you plan to wear the shirt outside, you spray your hair with antihumidity stuff before you leave the house, and two slices of bacon is enough 'cause you know I'm not giving up that bacon completely.

I want you to get in the habit of assessing yourself truthfully.

Absolute

We ask questions for only two reasons:
to get information and to stimulate thought.

It's true that these days, everyone seems to want to put a little label on you, tell you who you really are, and then put you on an endless path to self-improvement. Most of these self-appointed experts are so dull, so deadly serious—would it kill them to relax and smile? Because here's the living truth: self-assessment is not carved in stone, not always correct. A lighthearted look into your own heart is always better than a grim analysis. No one but you can really pinpoint you; only you know the real reasons for your relationships, your look, your successes and failures. And deep inside, not only do you know best where your weaknesses lie, you can spot them instantly, especially when you see them spread out on paper in a self-assessment exercise. And, no question, these go down easier when you approach them with a smile.

I consulted with the smartest people I know in the fields of health, psychology, self-improvement, and social interaction, and we've devised these quizzes and exercises to help you determine the areas in which you need work. No one's putting a label on you. No one even need see your answers, unless you choose to share them. These personal assessment inventories are throughout this book so you can test your own lifestyle. If you take them honestly, you'll get a fairly clear idea of your best and worst characteristics and the possibilities open to you as you go about becoming the best you can be. But you can also afford to have fun with them—take them by yourself or even with a friend, if you choose. Some of the questions might be lighthearted, but make no mistake, in the end they're serious business because if you're truthful, you'll gain interesting insights. That's a gift you can give yourself.

Chapter 2

How Healthy Are You, Really?

Avoid fried meats, which angry up the blood. If your stomach disputes you, lie down and pacify it with cool thoughts. . . . Go very light on the vices, such as carrying on in society. The social rumble ain't restful.

SATCHEL PAIGE ON HEALTH

If only that was all there was to it, Satchel. I found out the hard way how much more good health depends on than nonfried meats, cool thoughts, and going light on the vices. I'm lucky; I've enjoyed good health all my life, except for the few unpleasant show stoppers that pop up for almost everyone. My most serious health concern was my weight; it was undermining everything else—the way I felt, walked, played, not to mention the potential problem of heart disease waiting in the wings. It also, I was secretly sure, had something to do with the fact that although I always dated a lot, I still hadn't met the man who'd be my future. And because so many other women in this country grapple with too many pounds, I'm going to concentrate on weight almost exclusively in this chapter.

Let's start with my big gripe: I believe very strongly that in this country, we go from one extreme to another without batting an eye; it's just as easy to find a book that says, "Love yourself—no matter what size you are, you're wonderful," as it is to find a book that says, "If you're very obese, you're dying tomorrow." Well, it's very hard to love yourself when you don't fit in a bus seat, and by the same token, even if you're very obese, you're probably *not* dying tomorrow.

Absolute

Any truth taken to the extreme becomes error.

There never seems to be a middle ground that says we're talking about health here, not pounds. We recently had a discussion on *The View* about a new study that says many obesity dangers have been exaggerated in America. The study also said that people with a little heft are actually more healthy than very thin people. It may be true; I hope it's true.

But to their great shame, many in the food industry immediately seized upon the study to take out a big, stupid advertisement proclaiming that everything about obesity has been exaggerated and people should disregard everything they've ever read about obesity being unhealthy. Eat, eat, eat more was the implicit message. That's so unfair: self-serving advertisements like that only give people permission to eat excessively and be unhealthy. Look—overweight doesn't necessarily mean unhealthy, but obese means unhealthy, no matter how you cut it. Anorexic is unhealthy but, honey, so is obese. People hear what they want to believe. One doctor noted that when he advised people to drink a little red wine because it might help lower their cholesterol, they didn't hear the moderation part of the advice. All they heard was, "Drink wine—it's good for you." I know my own ears used to be clogged, if you know what I mean.

This is one of the reasons I won't advocate a particular weight-loss program. A full figure, a little heft, twenty extra pounds is not necessarily unhealthy for many, but there are some for whom—because of their heart, lungs, or blood pressure—those twenty pounds could be a matter of life or death. I have a girlfriend who during her pregnancy gained twenty pounds more than her obstetrician advised, and eight weeks before her due date, she had to be hospitalized because her blood pressure shot up wildly. For me, a few years ago, we weren't talking twenty pounds, we were talking more than a hundred pounds. My knees hurt, and I couldn't take a long walk. My chest hurt. I wasn't breathing properly—it sounded like I was gasping for air every time I opened my mouth. My back ached like mad. When I sat on a beach, I had to literally think about did I really have to go to the bathroom, because I knew I'd get so tired walking across the sand to get to the clubhouse restroom, then back to my place by the water. It was time to make a change.

I just didn't feel good. Until I didn't feel good, I always thought I was a fine-looking woman. Looking good to me has always been about the way I felt about myself. But as I started to feel crummier, I suddenly stopped looking good to myself and, I was sure, to everyone else. Then, the absolute worst happened. Shopping became hard work. I was in trouble. When I go to Paris with my favorite friends and I can't walk around the Place Vendôme, window-shopping, when I get too tired to go up and down the different floors of the Galeries Lafayette, changes must be made, okay? Changes must be made.

How Did She Lose All That Weight?

Now let me skip forward a minute. I am very conscious of the rumors and the gossip surrounding "how did she lose all that weight?"

I've purposely refrained from discussing the specifics of the weight-loss method that my doctors recommended for me because in all honesty, I don't want to be the poster child for any particular weight-loss method. So, "the Mouth from the South," as I've been called on occasion, refrained from talking about something that is about as clear as a big zit on your face: well, that seems to have made people all the more curious. So, here goes: I'm ready to tell you as much as I'm comfortable with, and I'll explain what makes me uncomfortable and why. Fair?

It seems to me that there are three recurring questions: why did she do it, what did she do, and why hasn't she talked about it?

Why did I do it? You already know. I felt lousy.

What did I do? First, I went to see several doctors, and I submitted to the most complete health assessment ever devised. Everything was checked—from my heart to my lungs, from my back to my ability to walk. I took stress tests, treadmill tests, cardiograms, X-rays, bloodwork—every test devised. Then, I sat down with my doctors to candidly assess my health. It wasn't a pretty picture. Although I didn't yet have any of the life-threatening ailments associated with morbid obesity, I was very much at risk of developing them. Ultimately, my doctors and I agreed that I needed to have complete medical intervention and supervision in a weight-loss program that would also be a long-term health plan. Long term? Try the rest of my life.

Why haven't I talked about it? It's really very simple. I had to figure out how I'd handle losing over a hundred pounds when I was in the public eye, daily. I would be naive to think people would not be interested. So, I started reading a whole bunch of magazine and newspaper articles about the hundreds of different weight-loss plans from pills to surgery, from the latest diets to food being delivered to your home. Gradually, I decided I wouldn't/couldn't be an advocate for any of them because I couldn't take the chance that someone who had a different body, with different problems, might follow the particular programs I chose but have a tragic result. Every weight-loss plan should have individual, tailored-for-you, medical advice behind it. Every serious weight-loss method has ups, downs, and sideways of risks, successes, and failures. A nonmedical professional can't know enough about your health to advise or recommend any method. Only your doctor can tell you what will work for you—just as my doctors told me what would work for me. I followed their advice to the letter, by the way.

There was something else. Born and raised in a loving but low-income family, I knew for a fact that not everyone has the resources to go about losing weight in the same way I did. Today, I can afford fantastic health insurance and also afford to supplement that insurance. I can afford to regularly consult a nutritionist, and I can afford to have my own cook weigh out my portions and prepare meals for me. I am enormously fortunate and blessed, and I know it. It would be disingenuous to say, "You too can do what I did and lose a hundred pounds," because unless you did every single thing I did, you might not get the same result. Great strides have been made in the area of weight loss, but some methods are still very dangerous, and although they have amazing results, they also can have tragic ones. Some weight-loss pills have heart ramifications; some diets greatly reduce the amount of carbohydrates, protein, iron, or calcium that your body may need; and some surgeries result in blood clots, infections, and even death. Only *you* and *your doctor* can assess what method will work with your body, your resources, your health, and your motivation.

It's Up to You—So, What Are You Gonna Do?

What I can do in this book is offer the very heart, the core of my long-term weight-loss plan because it can apply to everyone. That core is just good sense and can only be good. I'll share with you the three bottom-line principles of the way I changed my eating habits for the rest of my life. I deeply believe they are the only tried-and-true way that people ever really lose excess weight permanently.

The truth of the matter is that if you find yourself fat and not feeling well, you've got to do *something*. The prevalence of obesity in America is growing steadily and hitting everyone. Until recently, it was assumed that low-income people were the most at risk because in poor neighborhoods there tends to be more fast food and high-fat diets; healthy fare like fresh fruit is more expensive. Also, higher-income people have better access to education about health and more access to health care. But all that is changing.

A 2005 study reported by the American Heart Association concludes that the prevalence of obesity among Americans who earn more than $60,000 a year in family income is growing at a rate of three times higher than among their low-income neighbors. No one knows exactly why, but longer commutes, the growing popularity of restaurants, and longer work hours may play a big role, the researchers speculate. No one's immune. Americans are just getting fatter—all Americans, rich and poor. Here's a sobering statistic: at any given time, 15–35 percent of Americans are on a diet. No wonder: at any given time, 61 percent of American adults are either overweight or obese. Most of us are fat.

So, what are *you* going to do? If you want to prepare yourself for a healthy life (and a greater chance of love in that life), assess your physical health. Even though you haven't yet taken a battery of doctor-driven tests (eventually, you should) and gotten the medical expertise (you definitely should), you can still make a very general assessment of your physical well-being. Do it right now.

ASSESS YOUR PHYSICAL HEALTH

Respond to each statement with a number from 1 to 9. The more you believe the sentence describes you, the higher the number will be.

1. I am more than twenty or thirty pounds overweight. 1 2 3 4 5 6 7 8 9

2. I am more than fifty pounds overweight. 1 2 3 4 5 6 7 8 9

3. I am more than a hundred pounds overweight
(I have to shop in a specialty store or a large-size
department to find basic clothing). 1 2 3 4 5 6 7 8 9

4. I don't do enough exercise (minimum half hour,
three times a week). 1 2 3 4 5 6 7 8 9

5. Whether my body shows it in fat or not, I know
I eat too many really crappy things (you know a crappy
thing when you see it). 1 2 3 4 5 6 7 8 9

6. I usually eat whatever's around (candy bar? leftover
spare ribs? half a pastrami sandwich? several cups of
raisins? cold bacon strips?). 1 2 3 4 5 6 7 8 9

7. Most of the time, I eat take-out or fast food. Listen,
I'm a busy person. 1 2 3 4 5 6 7 8 9

8. Every day, I have a headache, backache,
teeth grinding, dizziness, stomach, or urinary problem.
It's always something. Otherwise, I'm fine. 1 2 3 4 5 6 7 8 9

9. I smoke or drink excessively (you know what
excessive means: be honest or don't bother assessing
yourself at all). 1 2 3 4 5 6 7 8 9

10. When I feel stress or fatigue, I pop a tranquilizer
or stimulant, either doctor- or self-prescribed. 1 2 3 4 5 6 7 8 9

11. I have one or more of the following: high blood pressure, high blood cholesterol, serious stress, frequent constipation, or diarrhea.   1 2 3 4 5 6 7 8 9

12. The next time I plan to have a complete checkup including a colonoscopy, chest X-ray, mammogram, or other appropriate diagnostic tool is probably *never*. Never works for me.   1 2 3 4 5 6 7 8 9

13. In the last year, I've been on at least one or two diets—and yo-yoed all over the place (lost weight, gained it back, lost weight, gained it back).   1 2 3 4 5 6 7 8 9

14. I sleep fitfully, terribly, sometimes not at all.   1 2 3 4 5 6 7 8 9

15. You want me to take a walk? Forget it. I take wheels or nothing.   1 2 3 4 5 6 7 8 9

ANSWERS AND ANALYSIS: Add Your Score

Did you score from 75 to 135?

Houston, we've got a problem. Good physical health rests largely on lifestyle choices—how much you move, what you eat, drink, smoke, or the pills you pop. I'm sure it will come as no shock to you that your health is in jeopardy according to accepted standards (no kidding around—this score is worrisome). With numbers at this level, you simply can't feel as well as you should, and your lifestyle is wearing you down; that's what happened to me before I vowed to change.

Face it: being obese certainly does put you at risk of developing serious medical conditions, not to mention exacerbating those you already have. Your score indicates you may have some issues in this department.

Even if you don't have serious weight problems, your physical assessment clearly indicates that you're doing something that doesn't love you, girl—only you know what it is. I don't know how to tell you this tactfully, so I'll just get it out: you have to make some serious adjustments in order to prepare yourself to be the best you can be, physically, let alone be ready to meet Mr. Right, or even Mr. Really Quite Good. Your score indicates a need for lifestyle changes in the health arena. One caveat: when you do finally make up your mind to get in good physical condition, speak to your doctor first. Then, don't opt for a crash diet or too vigorous an exercise regimen, which can do more harm than good. Unless you and your doctor decide that your health requires a more

continued

radical approach, it will serve you better in the long run to lose weight gradually—no more than 10 percent of your body weight over six months, says the American Heart Association. We're talking lifestyle here—the way you'll eat and exercise the rest of your life! It's not too late to reconstitute your health and appearance, and you know what? It's not even so hard—honest. I'll walk you through it. If I can do this, you can too. Right now, your score places you in a very dubious category—meaning, if you don't do something to change, I honestly can't figure out how you can be as happy as you deserve.

Did you score from 46 to 74?
Hmmm. Not terrible, sister, but far from great. You didn't need me to tell you that this is not an impressive score, although you're not walking on the brink . . . yet. While you seem to have a pretty sophisticated awareness of what makes for good health, your physical well-being is still not enough of a concern to you. Be careful. Respect your body more—don't feed it garbage and slothfulness. You're not doing that brilliantly, you don't look quite fine, because you're—well, I'd say kind of careless in the health department, when you could be shining, beautiful, and radiant with health. Take charge. Do the right thing, girl! Take the stairs instead of the elevator. Escalators don't count as stairs. Move yourself away from that TV and onto a treadmill. Throw out the cigarettes, now, this second, and never let them darken your health again. Eat better. Wear a seat belt in the car. You need more determination and commitment to achieve a really feel-good health style. Your score places you in a mediocre category; you know what you should be doing, you do it sometimes, but you're still pretty lax about your health, weight, and general fitness. C'mon—find your finest self!

Did you score from 30 to 45?
Less than fabuloso, but still, with a tad more self-searching and self-control, you're in a position to truly upgrade the physical part of your well-being. Listen—your score indicates that you do take reasonable care of yourself and appear to be in control of stress reactions. You like feeling and looking sharp, but you wish you felt that way more often. You love success. You know you're valuable. But even you can see room for lots of improvement—right? You probably don't often sabotage yourself—who doesn't stuff down a Whopper once in a while? Perhaps, it would be kind to say that you have quite a few too many "every once in a whiles." Still, you're pretty cool and your score places you in a potentially good position—not good Vanda, I said *potentially* good. With a little self-sharpening, you can easily move into the excellent category.

Did you score under 30?

Fabuloso. You're in the excellent category, honey, almost too good to be true—your score is wonderfully low. If you've answered the questions candidly and scored this well, you're definitely into health-making mode. It appears that you're healthy, you're strong, you're psyched and ready to meet your mate—or at least find love. A woman who cares for herself, respects her body, feels good, and presents a true picture of good health to the world, is primed to take on the world. Also, Denzel. Or Clive. Or Jimmy. Or Al.

But none of us is perfect. Check your assessments in the other areas of this book to see how you can come closer to perfection, not only physically but emotionally and spiritually.

*   *   *

How to Move into the Excellent Category

Here's the scoop from me, Star Jones Reynolds: in order to be all you can be physically, your body should be healthy and vigorous, and you really should live in that excellent category. You don't live there? I'll help you find your way home, but remember, I'm not going to advocate a particular weight-loss or exercise program because I'm not a nutritionist, nor am I a physician. Lawyers know about a lot about courtrooms and objecting, and zip about health regimens for others.

There are several popular methods to choose from that can be effective in jump-starting your healthy lifestyle change. Among them are:

* Peer group diets (e.g., Weight Watchers)
* Prepared food diets (e.g., Jenny Craig)
* Programmed eating diets (e.g., Atkins, the Zone)
* Appetite suppressants (medication)
* Surgical intervention (e.g., stomach stapling, banding)

Regardless of how any individual chooses to jump-start a weight-loss program, though, there are three things on which every doctor, nutritionist, health professional, and diet guru agree, and those three principles are what ultimately are working for me, long term. As far as I'm concerned, they comprise the only fail-safe diet in the world, the only one that works for most of us, and for the long run.

Are you ready? Write this down. Magic words.

Portion control
Nutritional balance
Exercise

Simple as that. Eat less. Eat right. Move more. In this country, we'll do almost anything to lose weight. I know someone who bought a bristle brush that would help her scrub away cellulite, and someone else who wore her magic weight-loss earrings everywhere: granted, these women aren't the sharpest knives in the drawer, but when you're desperate—hey, you'll try anything. But I, for one, am pretty fed up with diet crazes. You can take any diet on the planet—the low-carb diet, the high-carb diet, the South Beach Diet, the Scarsdale diet, the Weight Watchers diet, the Zone diet, the Three-Hour diet, the Dr. Perricone diet, the Atkins diet (Atkins Nutritionals filed for bankruptcy in August 2005), the French woman's diet, the ice cream diet, the grapefruit diet, the cabbage soup diet (that's right—*cabbage soup diet*): you name it, it exists. Think about this statistic: 95 percent of all dieters will regain their lost weight in one to five years. No surprises here: If any one of these really worked, why in the world would we be looking for yet another diet book? Wouldn't we all be on the same diet if it worked?

Rebecca Blake, MS, RD, CDN, is the senior dietician/nutritionist in the Department of Clinical Nutrition in New York City's Mount Sinai Hospital. She also runs the weight-loss program "Winning by Losing" at the fitness center in the famous 92nd Street Y in New York City, and she maintains a private nutrition counseling service. I'd say she knows a little about weight-loss plans that work.

"Portion control," says Rebecca, "is the major key to weight loss and its long-term maintenance. If you want to lose weight, you must not allow yourself unlimited portions of *anything*—except perhaps water. A diet like Atkins that promises you can eat as much as you want of X, Y, or Z is never optimal or beneficial for long-term weight loss. *Weight loss is about achieving a calorie deficit, and, as Star says, that's achieved primarily through portion control.* Period. The way you arrange for portion control is to consume fewer calories than you will burn by exercise. That ice cream diet, steak diet, bacon diet, cashew diet, or even cauliflower diet—whatever the promised 'miracle' food is this month—will never work long term because if you take too many calories in of any of these low-, high-, or no-carb foods, low-, high-, or no-fat foods, you will gain weight—that I promise.

"Still, I try not to even use the word *diet* when counseling my patients because it connotes hunger, deprivation, and other nasty things," says Rebecca. "Can you ever eat ice cream when you're on a weight-loss plan? Yes. What about that cupcake? Of course. You can eat everything in a healthy, balanced diet—the question is always, how much will you eat? That's portion control."

I'll say it again.

Portion control
Nutritional balance
Exercise

I had medical help *starting* my weight-loss effort but only discipline and these three elements will lead to my permanent healthy living. It works and it continues working. My guess is that it'll work for you. Of course, I can and will give you some of my own secret tips and my personal approaches to a firm, healthy body. I do believe that at this point, I'm eating and exercising in the most sensible and effective manner possible. It took me a long time, though, to get to the place where I was sure that what I put in my mouth and how I moved my body was the beginning of a process in which I could learn to love myself, and then love and be loved by a wonderful man.

If you feel you want to try one of those myriad diets I mentioned earlier, be my guest. It probably won't hurt you unless you go nuts. But in my experience, it will only work as a start to healthy living and will soon be abandoned. It's *always* not so much what you eat, but how much you eat that's the culprit. Also, human nature dictates that you can't stay on diets forever—they're pretty boring, and the moment you slip, you're on your way to gaining back whatever you lost. What I know works is the simplest plan in the world because it's more than a diet—it's a lifestyle change. You learn to eat intelligently and to exercise for the rest of your life. You don't need scales to measure your food, and you don't need books to figure out calories. All you need is common sense.

Best of all, you won't feel deprived. And when you meet the man of your dreams (when you're ready for him, naturally), he'll probably join you in a portion-control plan, not to mention a workout regimen.

Portion Control

I'm a firm believer in bigger is better for many things. Taxicabs, diamonds, and closets are all better when they're bigger. Food portions are not better when they're bigger. Overestimating what a reasonable serving consists of is probably the leading cause of obesity in America. Who makes up these portions? Insane chefs?

Here's what's not portion control:

* ※ A medium movie bag of popcorn: it contains sixteen cups of popcorn!
* ※ An average twenty-four-ounce steak at your local steak house: it contains six servings!
* ※ A pretzel from a street vendor: it's calorically equivalent to six bread slices, six one-ounce bags of pretzels, or eighteen cups of popcorn!

"I'm going to eat only one cookie," you decide. That sounds reasonable. The recommended serving size for a cookie is half an ounce. So, you go to the corner deli and buy only one cellophane-wrapped cookie—you wouldn't dream of being bad and buying a whole box of cookies. But the chocolate-chipper you've just purchased weighs about four ounces (about 700 percent bigger than the recommended cookie) and contains about 500 calories. Ever try leaving three-quarters of a cookie on your plate? Wouldn't happen. So, if the average adult female needs about 1,600 calories a day, do you really need to take up one-third of your whole daily calorie allowance with one cookie? You've been had. If a plate piled high with pasta and meat sauce will set you back 1,600 calories (and it will), is that all you're going to eat all day? Call that a portion?

Repeat after me: a serving is not a portion. A serving is the amount of food that nutritionists have decided is the standard amount of food that should be eaten by a healthy person, based on the calories it contains. A portion can vary in the number of servings on your plate. I've been in restaurants where I've received a plate (a portion) filled with four servings—and I can't believe I ate the whole thing. Felt no remorse. All I ate was one portion, right? No. I ate a humongous portion made up of four servings.

How Do You Know
When You Have a Reasonable Portion on Your Plate?

Throw out the calorie counter and use your eyes to measure "reasonable." For example, here are some measurements for which you do not need a scale:

* A potato: should be no bigger than your fist
* A portion-controlled serving of meat, fish, chicken, or pasta: the size of your palm, a deck of cards, or a computer mouse
* Half a cup of beans: a handful of beans
* A portion-controlled serving of French fries: about ten fries (a Wendy's Great Biggie gives you about a hundred fries—are they kidding?)
* A blueberry muffin: should be about 1.5 ounces (the size of an egg). A regular muffin from the corner deli is about seven times as big
* One serving of butter, margarine, or mayonnaise: the size of the tip of your thumb
* A chunk of cheese as an hors d'oeuvre: the size of four dice
* An apple: the size of a baseball
* One serving (one cup) milk, yogurt, or chopped fresh greens: a tennis ball
* Snacks (such as one serving of nuts or one-half serving of pretzels): can fit in one cupped palm
* A half-cup of veggies: can fit in one cupped palm
* One teaspoon of salad dressing: fits in the cap of a 16-ounce bottle of water
* One serving of cooked pasta: half a baseball

Bacon bacon bacon bacon bacon

You don't have to walk around with a tape measure to figure out what a controlled portion of food looks like. Mostly, you have to use your common sense. Portion control doesn't mean you have to eat what you hate—exactly the opposite. It just means you have to get in the habit of limiting what you love.

For example, my very favorite food in the whole world is bacon. You know how in some diets they ask if it would kill you if you couldn't have the one thing you really love? Yeah, it would kill me if I couldn't have bacon. I *love* bacon. I like turkey bacon, I like pork bacon. I like thick bacon, I like thin bacon. I'm like that little dog on television: "Bacon bacon bacon bacon bacon." I put bacon on baked potatoes, and I put it on an egg sandwich. Today, I had half a chicken club sandwich, and I put two strips of bacon on it.

Tricking Myself

Now, here's my biggest secret: I trick myself. Normally, two years ago, I would have four or five strips of bacon on that chicken club. Today—just two. It's a huge difference, but—guess what—I've come to the point where I don't even notice that I'm not chowing down on four or five strips. I do not deny myself my favorite thing in the whole world, but I limit it. I treat this change in lifestyle as a great victory because I don't want anyone, ever, to take away my bacon. I trick myself into thinking there are four slices on that sandwich, and because I've gotten so used to the two, it tastes and feels like four. By the way, on that chicken sandwich, I put a bit of low-fat mayonnaise on one side of the bread and nothing on the other (tricking myself into thinking there's mayonnaise on both sides). A vat of mayonnaise on the bread, incidentally, doesn't qualify as tricking yourself. Tomatoes, a slice of onion, some lettuce, and that bacon, and then the last step: *cut it in half* and only eat half. There's a great, portion-controlled chicken club.

If I could design my perfect dinner, this would be it: a portion-controlled steak, a satisfying half-plate of broccoli rabe, and a couple of tablespoons of mashed potatoes.

My perfect breakfast? Two strips of bacon and one scrambled egg with a little cheese (I don't have a cholesterol problem, so I allow myself this). No bread—although if I'm really hungry, I'll eat half a slice. Never, ever a bagel. Here's a little-known fact the bagel companies try to keep quiet: do you know that one bagel contains the calorie equivalent of five slices of bread?

Tonight, I'm going to have a portion-controlled piece of roast chicken: I'll put a whole chicken in the oven with some spices on it, bake it at 350 degrees, and in an hour, it's done. Then, I'll carve off my deck-of-cards portion (and put the rest away), add a spoonful of mashed potatoes, a lot of asparagus, and maybe a salad. What do I drink? More water than any human being ever drank. There are small bottles of water next to my bed in a small bedroom refrigerator. There are bottles of water in my living room and on my terrace. If you walk into my home, I'll offer you water first thing. It's not only a great weight-losing device, it's the best thing ever devised for gorgeous skin. Sometimes I'll drink diet root beer, sometimes grapefruit juice, but it's mostly water for this gal. Dessert? I'm the wrong person to ask on that. I don't really crave sweets. But if you crave, for example, giant chocolate-covered strawberries, have one giant chocolate-covered strawberry. One. That's portion control. I do admire oatmeal raisin cookies, so I'll have one or two after a meal a couple of times a month.

How Do You Know if You're Full?

Simple. I had to train myself to say, eat until you are full, Star, not until you are tired. If at the end of a meal you say something like, "That was sooo satisfying," you're full—not tired. But if you really feel more like saying, "Whew, Lord, I need to go lie down," you ate too much. This all translates into eat till you're no longer hungry, not till you're as bloated as the Michelin Man.

Ask Yourself, "Is It Worth All That?"

Say you need a dish of ice cream—you truly need it. You get up, go to the kitchen, put *one* scoop of ice cream in a dish, wash the spoon you used, put the ice cream back in the freezer, and walk away from the kitchen. Then you sit down to watch a television show or talk to friends. If you are so craving another scoop of ice cream, it means you have to get up from the television show you're watching or the friends with whom you're talking, go back to the kitchen, take the ice cream out of the refrigerator, get another spoon and a dish to put the ice cream in, and make yourself the extra portion.

Ask yourself, "Is it worth all that?"

If it's not worth it, you don't need that extra scoop, friend. And it's not.

What about Eating in a Restaurant with Friends: How Can You Control Portions?

This year, I had to host the international polo championships in Florida, and I invited my girlfriend Jaci along for the ride. We went to an Italian restaurant for dinner, and this is the way we ordered and ate. You can go out with your significant other, your girlfriend, or another couple and do it the same way. Everyone eats well and no one feels deprived. Jaci and I ordered one appetizer and one entrée for two of us. We knew we'd split everything. The appetizer was angel hair pasta with basil and chopped tomatoes in a light garlic sauce. The entrée was a veal chop. Both the pasta and the chop, as we guessed, were pretty substantial. In the old days, I would have ordered both the pasta and the veal chop (aren't you supposed to order an appetizer and an entrée? The restaurants hope you do) and scarfed down both by myself. But Jaci and I split the pasta and the chop. The meal was delicious and exactly what we wanted; when we finished, we felt satisfied and full but not tired.

Sometimes, when I go out with Al or friends, no one wants what I want, so there's no sharing. This is what I do: I order what I really want, and when it arrives, I cut it in half on my plate and send the rest back with the waiter to pack up right away. I eat slowly and appreciatively—I've learned to savor my food more when eating in this new way. I'm newly mindful of the flavor and texture of the food. Usually, half is enough when I'm not unmindfully gobbling down what's been placed in front of me. If I still feel hungry (and I can tell the difference now between being hungry and wanting to finish everything on my plate just because someone put it there), I'll wait for a few moments just to allow myself time to feel satiated and see if I'm really still hungry. I ask myself, am I hungry enough to open that take-out, have it re-heated, and brought back out to me? You know what? I have never opened the take-out to get another portion. Actually, I've gotten to the place where once I have it removed from the plate altogether, I'm not even tempted. Once you get used to eating controlled portions, anything else feels really excessive.

Number one truth: You have to get over the "children are starving elsewhere in the world" mentality.

Number two truth: When it comes to hunger, most of us are driven by what we see, not by how we feel. If too much food is placed in front of us, we'll come to perceive that it's a normal amount. If we get ourselves used to portion control, the smaller amount will seem far more normal than the whole, gigantic portion.

Number three truth: Controlled portions = discipline and true long-term weight loss; healthy living requires discipline, not compromise.

Star Tips

- If you're eating in a restaurant, ask for a doggie bag and silver foil right up front; when your food arrives, wrap half the amount and put it into the doggie bag right away. You can always take some out if you still feel hungry after eating what's on your plate—but I bet you won't. Now you have a nice lunch for the next day!
- Avoid buffets. It's almost impossible to practice portion control in an all-you-can-eat situation.
- For a while, until you're used to eating less, prepare portion-controlled meals in advance and then freeze them. You won't be tempted to go for that second helping if there is no second helping.
- Marinate foods in spices for flavor; foods that taste richly delicious (in flavor, not fat) make you feel more satisfied than bland offerings.
- Serve yourself (and your partner or guests) on individual plates, rather than in family-style, I'm-begging-you-to-take-seconds bowls.
- Never eat out of a bag or carton. Not even Chinese food.

⁕ Walk on by the door of a restaurant that promises supersize or jumbo portions. That restaurant doesn't love you.

*F*ast-food health? Nope—but maybe *healthier*. Live in the truth: fun is fast food; health is trail mix or a piece of fruit.

Still, I have to be fair here: some fast-food, supersize-portion restaurants, have seen the light, not to mention the loss of profit from more health-conscious customers. McDonald's, for example, started to feature "premium salads" consisting of warm breast of chicken—grilled or crispy (go grilled), Cobb salads, and fresh vegetables. Most restaurants in the Wendy's chain quickly followed suit with fresh fruit bowls, low-fat yogurts for dipping—and an option to switch a mandarin orange cup for the fries that usually come with a kid's meal. So, some fast-food restaurants do offer "healthier" choices.

But when I want to cheat, I cheat consciously. No piece of fruit's going to make me happy when I'm absolutely "Jonesing" for Micky D's. So, I confess, I occasionally have the burger—with a difference. I settle for the kiddie-meal cheeseburger and the kiddie-meal fries (the best French fries ever created in the history of the world but the most fattening in the universe—they must fry them in sugar and salt and everything that makes my life happy). I substitute a bottle of water for a soft drink. Now I'm satisfied. I've had my Micky D fix, but I've been smart enough not to do what I used to do: get the double quarter-pounder with cheese, extra mayo on the side.

⁕ Eat slowly. It takes about twenty minutes for your stomach to tell your brain you're full.
⁕ Sit down at a table while eating; pay attention to your food, tasting every bite. It's too easy to gorge mindlessly on French fries when you're lying in bed watching a Lifetime Original Movie.

I want to tell you something. Suppose, one day, you pig out on a double- or triple-size portion. Suppose you fall madly in love with a hot fudge sundae. No biggie. When it's over, it's over—put a lid on the guilt feelings. You didn't, as a friend of mine says, ruin your life or sell your baby on the black market. Get over it. Start back with your portion control the very next day. It's also helpful to try to figure out what contributed to your temporary lapse: Did you eat out of the carton? Did you have a really bad day? Were you stranded without food in the Sahara Desert for a week? What*everrr* . . . it's not the end of opting for portion control tomorrow.

Nutritional Balance

Mount Sinai Hospital's nutrition expert Rebecca Blake says that besides portion control and exercise, shooting for a nutritional balance in any weight-control plan is vital. If I didn't know that when I was obese, I sure know it now.

"You've got to choose foods from all the food groups to achieve a healthy nutritional balance," says Rebecca. "That's another reason why steak, cashew, ice cream, cabbage soup, and low- or high-carb diets not only don't work but are not healthy. We need *all* the nutrients, vitamins, and minerals that are found in dairy, protein, vegetable, fruit, and even fat food groups. Leave even one of these groups out, and the resulting food imbalance will render you nutritionally deprived and feeling unwell or fatigued. And for dating purposes, something even worse: people who follow low-carb diets, for example, complain of crankiness and something we call rancid fruit breath—not a terrific asset for meeting the love of your life. Does this mean you can't be a vegetarian and be healthy? Of course not. But, the vegetarian has to substitute other sources of protein such as tofu and soy products for the protein she's not getting from meat, chicken, or fish."

Balance. It's a good word. Avoid rancid fruit breath. Those are bad words.

Eat Only What You Love and Adore

I'm not a vegetarian, but I sure follow Rebecca's advice about substitution because there are many foods I don't like and I never eat them, no matter how great they're supposed to be for you. I hate and despise beets—don't put them anywhere on my plate. I hate cottage cheese—*ickh.* Anything that's squishy like Jell-O or raw oysters going down my mouth messes me up, uh-uh, I can't do it. I realize that I have to aim for nutritional balance, so I'll find substitutions that have nutrients similar to those in the icky stuff I despise. I love vegetables (except beets of course)—raw and cooked—and raw veggies make a great, nutritionally rich snack.

Ultimately, what is going to work for you in the weight-loss game is feeling satisfied. Modest portions of a variety of wonderful foods are the way to go. But you have to come to the point where you trust yourself enough to know that your body will tell you when it feels full. This takes some time to trust that body. In the old days, four years ago, I'd order a double Whopper with cheese and fries, eat the whole thing, feel stuffed, and think that was the normal way to feel full.

Snack Time

Everyone needs a handful of something to eat when reading or when watching some dumb television program. It's a good idea to prepare snacks in advance, so when you plop down on the couch to watch *Desperate Housewives* or *Girlfriends,* you'll reach for the good snack—not the Chunky Bar.

Some general thoughts on snacks:

* If you're eating something from a cellophane bag you bought in the supermarket, already I know you're in trouble. Chips? Pretzels? Just say no.
* A little protein mixed with a snack containing fiber makes you feel fuller. Try a half teaspoon of peanut butter on a piece of fruit, or top a whole wheat cracker with hummus. Mmmm.
* Peeled baby carrots sold ready to eat in a bag? A doll of a snack!

Try these other snacks: remember—take only one portion, and snack slowly.

* *Trail Mix*

> About 3 cups air-popped popcorn
> 3 cups unsalted pistachios, cashews, or walnuts
> 1½ cups Kashi cereal
> A few raisins
> 1 cup wheat nuts
> ⅓ cup sugarless dried blueberries

Mix, take a handful, and make it last. Put the rest away.

* *Dried fruit:* Raisins, for example, are healthy (low in sodium, fat-free), but the calories add up fast (about one calorie per raisin).
* *Fresh fruit:* I love plums. Love bananas. Grapes have a high water content, so they fill you up with a lot fewer calories than, say, raisins. Cut whatever you choose into small pieces and eat them languorously.
* *Fresh veggies:* Nothing like carrot, pepper, or celery sticks for snacking. Good and good for you.
* *Soy chips:* I hate to say it because soy is not my favorite thing in the whole world, but these tasty snacks have only about two-thirds the calories of potato chips and no saturated fat—and soy is good for you. But like anything else, they add up. Remember portion control: separate the bag of chips you buy into three or four little plastic bags and put three away for the next week.
* *Edamame:* Soybeans. This *is* my favorite snack (they don't taste like soy) and can be bought frozen, then defrosted in the microwave.
* *Veggie-based soup:* I love this when it's homemade. I freeze it in individual portions of one cup.

Some Final Thoughts on Food, My Mom, Weight Loss, Health, and Guilt

One of my favorite medical men is Dr. Andrew Weil, whose book *The Healthy Kitchen* (coauthored with Rosie Daley) is a mainstay in my kitchen. "Food is not the enemy," he declares in the introduction to the book, "and the dining table is not a minefield. I am unwilling to eat food that is boring, artless, and devoid of pleasure even if it's somebody else's idea of healthful."

Absolute

≈

Pleasure principle: Whatever pleases you once, you'll do again.

To that I say, amen. I love good food; trouble is, I loved it too much and I'd never heard of portion control.

My mom, who also never heard of portion control, never equated weight with looks, which was good and also terrible. I grew up in a home where fried foods seemed as healthy and natural as salads—it's that southern African-American thing. We sure were not overly health conscious. I mean, we would have salads and traditional southern vegetables—collard greens, string beans, and cabbage—but the veggies always had some sort of pork product mixed in, and the salads were heavy in delicious dressings. The good part was that I developed a taste that's more partial to real food than sweets and desserts, comforting food that makes you feel safe and good. My mom was always full figured, and she gained even more weight as I grew older. But the man I loved more than breathing, my stepfather, thought that she was sexy and beautiful and perfect just as she was. So, they were my role models. The good part of that is I watched how his eyes always followed her (and still do) when she crosses a room, and I grew up thinking that I was beautiful also, full-figured as I was. I had an image of what a man I loved thought was beautiful—and it wasn't skinny.

The bad part is that I didn't take care of my health as I should have, and my full figure turned into obesity. Today, I'm back to full figured. I'm never going to be skinny—it's just not my body and I will always have curves—but I will be healthy. I will never, ever again be unhealthy, tired, and weak because I haven't respected my body.

Here's a challenge for you: I ask that you do yourself a favor and stop buying into the fantasy version of the perfect body. The only perfect body is one that's healthy. Most of the fabulous pictures you see of those fabulous stars and models are airbrushed anyway—and I should know because mine are definitely airbrushed. Hey, I'm proud of my newly toned arms, but please, girl, they don't look that good!

If and when I have a daughter, I sure plan to teach her that the goal is healthy and happy—not skinny, not fat, not thin, not thick—physically, emotionally, and spiritually healthy. Period.

Full Figured vs. Fat

I hate confessions, but here we go:

There's a difference between being full figured and being fat. Once I was full figured (as I am now—just with less weight), but there came a time when I became fat. Out of shape, sloppy, morbidly obese, and not Star. I lost myself when I gained all that weight, and I went from the confident, happy, full-figured girl I loved being to the insecure, unhappy, self-conscious fat girl I didn't want to be. How do you know when you've crossed the line?

You know.

An Accident?

*P*erhaps it was an accident (but I don't think so) that I met Al when I'd lost about fifty pounds from "obese" and was in the process of losing even more. I think the Lord moves in mysterious ways, but this wasn't so mysterious: I was ready for love because I liked my body much more, and I felt so much better. People ask me how Al felt when I lost weight—don't forget he met me when I was still heavy. Well, he always encourages me to exercise for health. He'll say, for example, "Hey, girl, you're being lazy. I haven't seen you at the gym in a while." But in all our time together, he'd never commented on how I looked other than to say stuff like, "Oh, babe, you look great in that dress." But one

continued

day, I asked my husband the question people asked me—how did he feel about my weight loss? He thought for a bit and then for the first time he made a weight-related comment. He said, "It takes some getting used to—your thinner body beside me, because it's not the same body I fell in love with."

How sweet is that? About a week later, in bed, I said to him, "Honey, you have on your T-shirt—are you cold?" And he, whom most people consider to have one of the most gorgeous bodies on the planet—those shoulders—answered me by saying, "I just don't look as good naked as you do."

I thought to myself, "How did I find this guy?"

Exercise

At my heaviest, I never exercised. I don't know if it was because I was too tired to exercise because I was too fat, or just too tired, period. Whatever the reason for my couch-potato status, I knew I now had to start somewhere. Portion control and nutrition wasn't enough—I had to fine-tune the engine, firm up the chassis. Exercise would (the experts said) ensure the performance of my heart, lungs, muscles, and increase flexibility (not to mention the look of my flabby upper arms); it also would have an effect on my emotional readiness for a partner.

I did know a little about exercise, as you all do. You'd have to be living in a box not to have heard of the advantages of aerobic fitness and weight lifting. I knew that cardiovascular exercise would help my ability to deliver oxygen and nutrients to tissues, heart, and lungs; it would also keep my blood pressure low and help with weight loss. I knew that I needed strong, toned muscles and body flexibility to continue working and walking (and don't forget shopping) at the pace I chose. Even my posture wasn't terrific. I had to get moving.

There are always one or two straws that break the proverbial camel's back, that make you say, Okay—this is it. I'm not going to take it anymore—I'm taking charge. I had those straws. Three straws, to be exact.

The first straw had to do with my asthma inhaler. I did not want to use that damn inhaler. First of all, and I know this is the vainest reason in the world, when I went out in the evening, the thing took up too much space in my small purse. I did not want to have that asthma inhaler in that space. I had one in the car, one at work, one next to my bed, and I hated them all. But I had to have the rotten things. Once, in Aspen, I couldn't breathe and I truly panicked. My blood oxygen level went down to 60 (that ain't terrific). So, breathing was a huge health goal for me and a reason I started to exercise. (Let me jump ahead for a second and say that as I write this, it's been over two years since I've used or carried an asthma inhaler.)

The second straw that drove me to exercise was the ability to cross my legs. I didn't have it. I'm not talking about looking good crossing my legs, oh no, darling, I'm talking about being able to physically do it at all. When I sat, I was uncomfortable, and I felt all squished up with too tight clothes and unsupple limbs. Jumping ahead again—the day I finally crossed my legs, I was home talking to someone, and without thinking, I just crossed my legs. I looked down—crossed legs! Whoa!!!!!!!!

The third straw? I wanted to be able to put on my own necklace. When you're heavy, to stretch your arms out with your elbows at right angles to your body and keep your arms up there while you fasten your necklace is hard.

I put on my own necklace now.

So, I faced the truth: any weight-loss plan had to include exercise.

Let's talk about general exercise and goals in a minute. I want to tell you what I personally did to start moving my body properly and healthfully.

Dealing with the Doctor

The first thing I did before I started my dieting or exercise program was to see my doctor. You know I've read this a million times: talk to your doctor. But what do you *say* to your doctor? No one ever tells you that. Perhaps a few specifics on what to discuss with your doctor regarding weight loss might be in order, right here. Dr. Nieca Goldberg, spokesperson for the American Heart Association and chief of the Women's Heart Program at Lenox Hill Hospital in New York City, suggests you write down the following list of *general* things to discuss with your doctor; certainly, take the list with you to your appointment to talk about an exercise plan, if one is prescribed. Tell the doctor about:

* Your health concerns
* Symptoms you've noticed
* Past illnesses and medications
* Family history of heart disease and other illnesses
* Medications you're taking (and have taken in the past)
* Your lifestyle habits—diet, smoking, past exercise (in my case, this was zero exercise)
* Causes of stress in your life
* What you want to accomplish with exercise

My own primary doctor on the team involved in my weight-loss plan suggests this conversation to have with yourself, then with a physician:

First ask yourself: Is my weight really a problem? Can I get around, is personal hygiene difficult, am I short of breath if I walk a couple of blocks or even one flight of stairs? If you acknowledge you have a problem, then ask the doctor the following *specific* questions:

* What methods of weight loss are you familiar with—a low-fat diet, a high-protein diet, portion control, etc. What have your other patients done that is successful?
* What are the resources you have available to help me on my journey? For example, is there a nutritionist on your staff? Are there personal trainers on your staff? (Usually, only weight-loss specialists will have these "perks.")
* How do I know if I'm unhealthily obese or just fat? Until recently, doctors measured a person's fat by a mathematical formula called a Body Mass Index. If your weight in kilograms divided by your height—in meters squared—exceeded 30, you were seriously obese.

    There's a better way to judge, according to a new worldwide study of 27,000 people reported in the prestigious *Lancet Medical Journal*. This cutting-edge test of unhealthy obesity considers where your fat is located—not just how much fat you have. Why? Fat stored around the waist is more likely to clog arteries than fat stored around the thighs and hips. The new test uses the ratio of waist size divided by hip circumference. The danger point for cardiovascular risk is more than 0.85 for women and 0.90 for men. Bottom line: a larger waist line than a hip line is bad news when predicting health problems, especially heart attacks. Your doctor and many Internet sites can determine your hip-to-waist-size ratio.

Sometimes, the doctor you consult will refer you to a weight-loss specialist called a bariotritionist. That specialist might discuss the various methods of weight loss that are available.

Bring a notepad or paper to any appointments (or even a small tape recorder) so you can go over the doctor's responses later, when you're not nervous.

So, I spoke to my doctors. And they spoke back to me—about exercise.

My Exercise Routine

After discussions with doctors, my own research, and checking out my thinking with my best friends, I hit upon the plan which would work best for me. It changed my life, that's all. Each person must experiment to find the type of exercise she likes. It will work for her because if she likes it, she'll do it.

You might have heard of my personal choice; it's called **Pilates.**

The Pilates phenomenon has been catching on in most parts of this country, not to mention Canada, Europe, and even Asia. It's a method of exercise created to balance, stretch, tone, and strengthen the body. Designed by a boxer and a performer named Joseph Pilates around 1914, it involves equipment that incorporates spring tension, straps to hold feet or hands, and supports for the back, neck, and shoulders. There are more than five hundred controlled, precise movements, and the exercises require concentration, as you might guess. Pilates also encourages mat work, which is exercises done on the floor. Joseph Pilates believed that consistent deep breathing was integral to good, strong lungs and bodies. He believed that strengthening what he called the "power-house"—the muscles of the lower abdomen, lower back, buttocks, and pelvic floor were the source of great health and a firm, trim body.

Strength and flexibility (particularly of the abdomen and back muscles) are a big Pilates goal. Keeping the spine in neutral alignment works deep muscles safely even as it protects against back pain. Muscular and emotional coordination are integral to the program, which promises (and delivers) great posture and balance, increased bone density, and joint health, not to mention stress reduction. Don't be put off by the fact the machines have names—sometimes scary ones like the Reformer. Another is the Cadillac, and yet another is the Wunda Chair. You really need an instructor, at least in the beginning, to conquer the Reformer.

I love it. It's a great way to tone and slim troublesome spots like waist, hips, upper arms, and thighs. I needed that.

Here's the bad news: it can get pretty pricey. I do my Pilates three to four times a week in a Pilates studio with special Pilates trainers Julie Rose of Power Pilates and Lesa Salvano of In Balance Studio. A less expensive way to do it is to join one of the myriad gyms that offer Pilates along with other kinds of exercise equipment, including, perhaps, a pool; the Pilates classes usually come along with the price of yearly membership.

General Exercise

Let's talk general exercise: *the best exercise is the one you'll do,* and I need to be motivated and definitely not bored. Again, I went back to my doctor to ask her to recommend something that would step up my exercise program but still give me a Pilates experience. Her suggestion? **Core Fusion.** If Pilates changed my life, Core Fusion at the Exhale spa is helping me live it to the fullest.

Core Fusion, developed by Elisabeth Halfpapp and Fred DeVito, is a tightly choreographed fitness class that flows from weight work to ballet-based moves to exercises that borrow from Pilates, yoga, and orthopedic smarts. It's geared toward strengthening your core—the area between your butt and your abs—but believe me, every part of my body feels stretched and buffed when I finish a workout. Core Fusion is actually a mind-body class in many ways because a sense of peace and relaxation accompanies the resulting long, lean muscles and more flexible body. A tough but wholly efficient workout—I love it.

Finally, I have also gone the route (and still do, sporadically) of general exercise, and that can work wonderfully if your main priority is to keep at it. This is what I now know about exercise in general:

Small goals

Whatever exercise you choose, make sure you've got a realistic plan. If you've never worked out in your life and then say you're going to go to the gym five days a week for the rest of your life, you should know your plan is ridiculous and dumb—because you're not going to show up. If you make unrealistic goals, you're going to set yourself up and get all geeked up and be excited the first two or three days. And then you're going to stop. And you're going to be frustrated. And then you're going to eat. Not good—okay?

So, I make what I like to call small goals. During the eight weeks before my wedding, when my mission was to weigh less than Al on that day, I did intensive boot camp workouts with four different trainers in addition to Pilates. Four trainers every week, five days a week for eight straight weeks! It was crazy, it was nuts, I was working my rear end off because I wanted to meet that goal. But it was a very short-term goal—and I was determined to meet it. I managed but I couldn't maintain it now if I wanted to: the goal is no longer there, but the discipline it took to reach it is and will be for the rest of my life.

It helped that as I started, Suzanne, my lead trainer at "E," the Equinox elite training facility, said to me, "Your only goal is to get here. If you get here, I'll do the rest."

So, my first goal was simply to get up and get to the gym. After I attained my wedding weight, I set even smaller goals. If I did nothing else, I would not take the elevator but walk up and down seven flights in my building every Monday. Then, my goal was to walk the stairs Mondays and Wednesdays. My next goal was to walk up and down the stairs two days a week and take a class a week at the gym. Then, I moved from one weekly class to two classes.

Take very tiny steps in your exercise program. Move yourself into good health at a slow pace. As you accomplish each short-term goal, you're excited to add a new one.

What Your Exercise Program Should Be Doing for You

You've made the realistic plan. You've decided where you want to be in three months, and you got there. Your exercise program should now provide you with cross-training—a little of everything.

Want to feel stronger? Want to feel less pain and stiffness, and more suppleness? Do you want to see that flabby skin get firmer and more attractive? Want to get closer to loving yourself—and thus making yourself more attractive to Mr. Terrific, who's waiting on the sidelines somewhere? Go, girl. If you belong to a gym, ask the trainers to help you set up a balanced and realistic cross-training program. If you're exercising on your own, the all-around exercises should include:

- **Cardiovascular training.** Aerobic activities like running, walking, biking, and swimming strengthen the heart, lungs, and muscles. An aerobic activity should elevate your heart rate and maintain that elevation for at least twenty minutes. Getting on that treadmill is no longer a matter of losing weight for me: it's a matter of living in health. It's a matter of being able to take a long walk on the beach without panting with frustration.
- **Bone strengthening.** The treadmill and careful training involving weight-lifting, cables, push-ups, and other resistance activities help muscles as well as bones become stronger.
- **Flexibility training.** Muscle inflexibility can restrict the back's ability to move, rotate, and bend. Stretches and exercises given under Pilates, tai chi, and yoga make you supple and flexible.

Do It on the Net

Okay—you say you're just too busy to go anywhere to exercise, and maybe you don't have the funds to get a personal trainer to come to you. A recent article in the *Wall Street Journal* caught my eye because it outlined something very different—"high-tech" workouts that sounded just great! The article maintained that your most effective piece of home exercise equipment may be your computer. On the Web, anyone can now gain access to specialized trainers at highly reduced prices compared to a regular gym or a pricey personal trainer. Online personal training sessions usually involve one-on-one contact with exercise experts or trainers similar to those you'd get at a gym—but it's all by e-mail. Exercise guru Bob Greene, for example, Oprah Winfrey's personal trainer, offers self-contained, online training classes.

The low price for online training is the big plus: a regular personal training session can cost anywhere from $50 to $100 an hour, but many online training sessions cost as little as $5 to $10 a week. The added bonus is that you don't have to schedule appointments or fight traffic to get to the gym.

Does it work? You must be the judge if it works for you, but a 2005 study published in the *Journal of the American Medical Association* says it definitely produces results; another study from Brown University says the same.

Some caveats, notes the *Journal:* ask questions to determine whether you're really getting personal feedback from a trainer or just from an assistant or a prepackaged program (which may or may not also be effective). You might also look for certification from the American College of Sports Medicine (acsm.org), the American Council on Exercise (acefitness.org), or the National Strength and Conditioning Association (nsca-lift.org). Here are some suggestions for Web fitness programs:

1. Jeffgalloway.com (personal e-mail coaching from an Olympic runner)
2. Markallenonline.com (a triathlon trainer who is an Ironman champion)
3. Cardiocoach.com (these are coached workouts and music on CDs)

4. Totalbodymakeover.com (this is Bob Greene's site for his prepackaged twelve-week book course, but Oprah's trainer also will be offering personal training early in 2006). Click on Bob@eDiets to get to his online program.

Remember: You can't do all the exercises, all the time. You can do some of them, some of the time.

Excuses

Bottom line: exercise has to be one of those life activities you do without questioning it—even when you're not in the mood, like brushing your teeth and taking a shower. But I know you—you're like me—you're going to try to trick yourself out of exercise with an excuse. Here are some of the more popular ones:

* *Popular Excuses for Avoiding Exercise (with apologies to the Seven Dwarfs)*

I'd exercise but I'm . . .
Too sneezy
Too grumpy
Too dopey
Too bashful
Too sleepy
Too happy
Too busy
Too achy
Too old
Too depressed

Excuses rejected. Start moving. *Hi ho, hi ho, it's off to gym I go* . . . Cute, right? Well, maybe not so cute. Still, I'm not going to let you off that easy.

The following excuses are probably closer to what you really say—and here's what *I* say to you.

* **I have no time.** You have time to do everything else: manicure, gossip on the phone, go to the sale at TJ Maxx. . . . Come on, girl, I've used this one.

* **I'm too tired.** It's because you're overweight. A large amount of weight makes you lethargic and lazy. I was so lazy, I once had a golf cart drive me from one end of the studio to another when I was shooting a commercial. I said I was too tired to walk, but I was actually too heavy to move comfortably without sweating off my makeup.

* **I'm embarrassed.** Who you telling! Your butt is bigger than those other women and so what. You aren't doing it for them, you are doing it for you. Yep, people will be mean and nasty, they will say things to hurt your feelings, but you have a goal—to get healthy. Let me tell you, girl, the first time you bend over and your spandex pants droop not because you stretched them out, but because you need a 1X instead of a 2X—it's like manna from heaven.

* **I'm afraid of the atmosphere.** Gyms can be intimidating. So, don't go to one that is a breeding ground for "muscle heads" and "ballet dancers." Also, take your favorite motivational tape or music, and tune in the positive and tune out the negative.

* **I don't know what to do at a gym.** Real concern. Along with almost every new gym membership you sign comes a few sessions with a trainer who will walk you through the machines, the facilities, and the classes offered. Take advantage of the overview and then try to use a trainer at least once a week to keep you on the right track, and change up your routine even if it costs a little extra.

* **I have no one to go to the gym with.** So? Again, it's not about them, it's about you. When you hear of the greatest shoe sale on the planet— I'm talking $9.99 for everything in the store—you don't wait for a partner.

* **I'm self-conscious about the way I look.** Focus on the way you feel. I didn't see how bad I was looking till I started to really *feel* bad. How

does your body feel? The moment your body feels better, I guarantee you will look better. If nothing else, it will put a smile on your face, and that already makes you prettier.

An Interesting Finding

A few years ago, Harvard University released the results of a fifty-year land-mark study of the factors that go into a happier life. The study was reported in a book called *Aging Well,* and it offered the top seven factors that predict healthy aging. Not surprisingly, regular exercise figured prominently among those seven factors. The study also found that exercise is easier and more enjoyable with a partner, although *not* having a partner is not a good excuse for avoiding exercise. When you meet Mr. Right, he could be your jogging partner—something to look forward to. Check back in three months with me to see where you are. I'm still working hard at it, so let's do it together. Let me know your successes and your failures. Let me know how you feel—e-mail me at www.Star Jones.com and I'll be your partner!

A Not-So-Pretty Finding

This may not be the right note on which to end this section, but it has to be said.

I hate to be the bearer of bad news, but the truth shall set ye free: not everyone wants you to be slim, trim, healthy, and happy. I think there's some faulty psychological dynamic that tells some people they can vent their hidden rages, their own insecurities, even their too virtuous pity on fat people. When you hear people in the media or even acquaintances making fat jokes, you know it's because something in them feels more strong and victorious if they have scapegoats to pick on. Fat people are their anger outlet. You hear the fat anger from mean-spirited media people, and you might even hear subtle antifat comments in your own circle of acquaintances. But what you never expected is anger directed at you because you lost weight!

You know what? You *will* hear this from some you thought were friends.

We recently had two young women on *The View* who were the subject of a 2005 *New York* magazine article called "Suddenly Skinny." Both of these young women had undergone some sort of weight-loss surgery. Both of them were really health oriented because they had been ill from their excess poundage. One woman had a knee replacement in her future if she didn't lose the weight, and good-bye to her job as an active police officer. The other woman had been big all her life, and her mother had died from complications of obesity. She also knew that she was on a path to trouble.

One of the young women was very, very attractive. She had this really beautiful face, a gorgeous smile, and long, luscious hair. But she never embraced how pretty she was, and she didn't live her life like "I'm a pretty girl." When she finally lost weight, her confidence zoomed up—that often happens. But inexplicably to some, she revealed on our show that a number of her friends stopped speaking to her or simply weren't nice to her anymore.

One of my gorgeous, always-has-been-slim cohosts asked in amazement, "But why would that happen?"

I knew why. I've been there, done it. So, I piped in and said, "They've turned on you, Miss Marie, because they were more comfortable putting you in the fat, lonely, and single category and box for the rest of your life. They would have been happy with that."

"Absolutely correct!" said our guest.

So, this is what I have to tell you: very few things are universal with people who've lost weight, but that experience is universal.

Absolute

Never allow anyone to place a period in your life.
Control the punctuation—it's your life.

You will have lots of people who are happy for you and excited and really just want the best for you. One of my biggest cheerleaders, for example, has been my girlfriend the actress Vivica A. Fox. Vivica is considered one of the most beautiful women in America. I'm telling you there's not a week that goes by that she doesn't call me to say, "Girl, you was lookin' good on the show today. You lookin' hot, mama. Go ahead. You better go." She's always just very encouraging, and even when I was the fat girl in the group, she was the same.

Still, when I was heavier, she would worry a lot, but even then, she would say something like, "Okay, Star, what's happening now—you okay?" She wasn't on me, she didn't say, "You need to diet, you need to do this, you need to do that," but she also didn't ignore it when she knew I was struggling with being overweight. It wasn't in the back of her head every moment. It wasn't something that she threw up in my face, but she often acknowledged her worry in her way. And as I began losing weight and taking better care of myself, she acknowledged that also. And now she is simply joyful to see me healthy and happy.

You've got the "Vivica" friend—I know you do—but you will also have the other kind of friend or acquaintance—the kind who secretly doesn't wish you well because she needs a victim, she needs someone who has it worse than she does, and when you were fat, you were that victim for her. Or him. Do not expect this person to be thrilled that you were victorious in your efforts.

Rise above! Revel in your new body and new opportunities. Delight in your ability to prepare yourself physically for a new life. Embrace your true friends. Lose the others.

Shine!

Chapter 3

Are You Your Most Gorgeous?
Fashion, Makeup, and Hair

The world is governed more by appearance than realities.

DANIEL WEBSTER

Trying to be physically healthier has to start with the health of your body. But make no mistake, girl, after health, after the dropping of the pounds, you have to feel physically better in other important ways—like feeling pretty. *Pretty* is a magical word. It brings confidence and wit and self-esteem. You walk pretty and you talk pretty when you feel pretty. If the grand love of your life just happens to be walking behind you into the Beyoncé concert tomorrow, will he be dazzled by your pretty hair, your pretty face, your pretty dress? Are you lookin' good, Cassandra? Will your style stop him dead in his tracks?

When all is said and done, we want to be remembered for our style—our very best look. But outward style is no more than a presentation of self—our inner selves, our adorable selves, our most convincing selves. Sure, we all have those three-o'clock-in-the-morning moments when we feel plain, klutzy, unattractive, but the true stylist will wake up in the morning, pick out her cutest outfit, and powder, brush, dress, and color the best parts of her *self* to come shining back. Intelligence makes you unforgettable, manners and tone of voice make you interesting and appealing, but the best presentation of the physical you makes you irresistible.

Be your most gorgeous. Don't for a moment think that strong women have to be all hard angles and unfeminine. That's the biggest mistake people make about women who change the world: the forceful, funny, most delightfully convincing women usually look terrific, and they are adorable.

Before I let loose with my feelings about looking wonderful, take the general beauty assessment below. It concentrates not on any one aspect but on your general habits and feelings about your appearance. Then we'll talk.

ASSESS YOUR LOOK

Choose the answer that best describes you:

1. This is how I mostly feel about shopping:

A. I'm out of my element in a clothing store, and choosing the right accessories seriously frightens me. I was okay when everything had to match, but they changed the rules!
B. I choose clothes that are baggy, gappy, flowing, BIG, because that hides my fat. The last time I wore a shirt tucked in, I was eleven.
C. Love it. I spend more money than I can afford.
D. Love it. I know how to play the game.

2. I'm happiest in

A. Supercute track pants and a T-shirt
B. Oversize jeans—comfort is all
C. Designer anythings
D. Dress-up, chicly styled clothing
E. Pj's

3. Love these accessories:

A. Large hoop earrings
B. Real gold or platinum jewelry
C. Funky stuff
D. Whatever's hot
E. I rarely wear accessories

4. If I could raid a celebrity's closet, I choose

A. Beyoncé
B. Paris Hilton
C. Anna Kournikova
D. Diane Keaton
E. Nicole Kidman
F. None of the above—I choose my own closet

5. What words do you often hear?

A. You have such a pretty face, but . . .
B. I only tell you because I love you, but you really ought to go for a makeover/lose some weight/do something with that hair.
C. Where did you get that incredible shirt/hat/dress/purse?
D. You have some schmutz on your shirt, *there* . . .

6. You shop

A. At the end of the season when the sales come
B. Hardly ever
C. At outlets
D. At the start of the new season when you know what's "in" and you can get a lot of wear from the clothes you buy

7. When was the last time you bought into a popular trend?

A. When grunge was popular.
B. I don't buy trends—I buy what looks good on me, and I try to find it on sale.
C. The last trend—what was it? I love to be trendy.

continued

8. If you haven't changed your look in five years, why?

A. I look good just the way I am.
B. I have better things to do than worry about my look.
C. I don't know where to start.
D. No time, no money.
E. I do change my look occasionally.

9. When you dress up, you generally feel

A. Klutzy and unpretty
B. Very appealing, maybe even adorable, maybe stunning
C. I almost never dress up
D. Just all right, passable

10. When you see friends who haven't seen you lately, they often say something like

A. "You look exactly like you looked in high school/college."
B. Nothing. They usually don't comment on my looks.
C. "You've changed—you look fabulous!"
D. "Who does your hair?" or "What color lipstick is that?"

11. You catch your reflection in a passing mirror. Your first thought:

A. Arrrrrrgh
B. Boring
C. Ooooh—lookin' good

FACT OR FANCY?

You may have heard some of these are true from your best friend, you've always *thought* some were true—but were you correct? Check your fashion savvy. Are the following statements fact or fancy?

12. Circle the right answer for each

A. Don't mix patterns: stripes and plaid, yeccch.	FACT	FANCY
B. Man-made fabrics (polyester, rayon) scream tacky.	FACT	FANCY
C. Fake jewelry screams cheap. Better one good, real piece than five costume jewelry reproductions.	FACT	FANCY
D. High heels give you a sense of power.	FACT	FANCY
E. On miniskirts: age doesn't figure in. If you have a good figure, wear them.	FACT	FANCY
F. Buy cheap—duplicate expensive.	FACT	FANCY
G. Classic is best. Throw out the ruffles.	FACT	FANCY
H. Your purse and shoes should match—even if nothing else does.	FACT	FANCY

13. Where do you most often get your inspiration for your look?

A. *Sex and the City* and the fashion catwalks

B. Your mom

C. Old movies

D. Magazines

E. Stuff you see at the mall

F. Women on the street who have a very individual look

14. How long does it take you to get ready for a big date or an important occasion?

A. Somewhat under an hour

B. Ten to twenty minutes

C. Between an hour and a half and two hours

15. If you could pick your body type it would be

A. The bod I own—I like it

B. Curvy and full—like a Rubenesque beauty

C. Toned, muscular, and athletic

D. Thin, thin, ultrathin, Nicole Richie thin

continued

ON MAKEUP

16. My approach is

A. Minimal: I rarely wear any makeup products.

B. Maximum: I try everything new—I love experimenting!

C. Scattered: I wear whatever's in my medicine cabinet.

D. Selective: I buy good but primarily inexpensive brands.

E. Pricey: You get what you pay for—I buy only superior name brands.

17. About my face: I feel

A. Confident when I bop along the avenue

B. Very plain

C. God—I should have looked in a magnifying mirror before I left the house

D. Cheated

18. Killer makeup is

A. Usually subtle—sometimes you can't even see it

B. Individual—usually different for you than for anyone else

C. Expensive—get what you pay for

D. Cheap—smart money rules

E. All of the above

F. None of the above

19. You've used up a tube of lipstick

A. Never. In fact, many of your lipsticks have not even been opened.

B. A million times. You're loyal to your favorite shade.

C. Rarely.

20. About how many lipsticks do you own?

A. About 2

B. About 25

C. About 8–10

21. Tomorrow looks like a beautiful day! You'll be

A. Watching *Who Wants To Be A Millionaire.*

B. Lying down in an avocado-oatmeal mask, tweezers in one hand, moisturizer in another.

C. Pulling on your navy blue jeans. You're out of here—eyebrows and skin can wait.

D. Taking this beauty quiz.

22. The guy you've been digging on asked you out to a last-minute movie which starts in ten minutes. You're not dressed yet. Will you be ready in time?

A. No sweat. All you plan to do is spray a little deodorant on the important parts, anyway.

B. You need twenty minutes, max. At least you'll make it before the trailers finish.

C. Arghhhhhh. You'll miss this flick because you need over an hour to get your "beat" on.

23. Beauty product you can't live without?

A. None. I don't really wear makeup.

B. Lip gloss and blusher—I need that shimmery glow.

C. Anything glittery—I like to sparkle like a star.

D. I can live without any particular product: can always find an alternative.

24. It's the day before your best friend's party, and a big zit has emerged on your nose. You:

A. Squeeze it

B. Ignore it and have a good time

C. Buy some miracle lotion and treat that puppy!

ON HAIR

25. Your hairstylist

A. Suggests little variations every time you visit—a little highlighting here, a little layering there, a few wisps, a sleek look.

B. Can read your mind, which isn't too hard because you've worn the same hairstyle for years.

C. Is the source of all gossip and the best doctors and knows every personal detail of your life.

D. Seems to regularly disappoint you—but you understand that he can't make a silk purse out of a sow's ear.

continued

26. My hair is

A. An accessory—I change it as often as I do my earrings
B. Too dull, too curly, too mousy, too thin, too straight, too something
C. Fabulous
D. Miserable to manage—I hate spending time on it

27. If you were half an hour late waking up for work or school, how would you cut corners to get there on time?

A. Wear my hair rollers under a scarf on the way—then brush out as I arrive.
B. Refuse to rush, and get that hair *right*. I'm not compulsive about arriving exactly on time, so I'd take my usual hour to prepare: appearance is key.
C. Leap up, pull my hair back, brush my teeth, and leave (after a quick glance in the mirror).

28. How would you describe your daily hair routine?

A. Wash and wear—brushing optional. No fuss, no muss.
B. Wash, condition, set, blow dry, style.
C. Killing, aggravating, time-consuming. Hate it.
D. I experiment: sometimes a shampoo and blow dry; sometimes simply a hair weave or wig. Whatever—I rarely go for the same look. I'm a mix-and-match momma.

29. My favorite hair secret

A. Hair accessories: faux fur ponytail holder, great barrettes, big tie-back clips, pretty scarves.
B. One hundred brush strokes daily
C. Hair spray—couldn't live without it
D. I adore experimenting with color

30. You've just been swimming when—oh no—no hairbrush. What to do?

A. Nothing. No one will notice because your hair is always messy, anyway.
B. Luckily, you keep a funky hat in your bag for emergencies.
C. Borrow a hat (or brush) from friends. Messy hair is not you.

SCORING AND ANALYSIS

Score as directed, then add the result.

1. A=0, B=0, C=3, D=10 (It *is* a game!)

2. A=10, B=2, C=4, D=10, E=0 (An A or D answer indicates that you know what you like; the other choices indicate insecurity.)

3. A=8, B=10 (can never go wrong), C=5, D=8, E=0

4. A=3, B=3, C=3, D=3, E=3, F=10 (Their closets may hold insanity—only your choices count as fashion that makes you feel good.)

5. A=2, B=0, C=10, D=0

6. A=8, B=0, C=10 (my way!), D=6 (And you'll pay top dollar.)

7. A=0 (You opted for absolute ugly), B=10, C=2

8. A=6 (maybe your self-esteem is fine, but are you sure you're not avoiding change?), B=0, C=0, D=0, E=10

9. A=0, B=10, C=4, D=2

10. A=4 (unless you looked smashing then, in which case take 10), B=0, C or D=10

11. A=0, B=0, C=10

12. A, B, C, E, G, H=FANCY. D and F=FACT. Take 2 for each correct answer you marked.

13. A=6, B=4 (unless your mom dresses like Halle Berry), C=2, D=8, E=0, F=10

14. A=10, B=3 (You're not paying attention, Kendra), C=0

15. A=10, B=6, C=6, D=2 (Anything other than A indicates you're not satisfied with your body today and must work on your physical presentation.)

16. A=1, B=1 (you're a makeup junkie!), C=0, D=10, E=4

17. A=10, B=0, C=0, D=0

18. A=5, B=5, C=5, D=5, E=10 (This is the only one that rings true because makeup always depends on your mood and the occasion), F=0

19. A=2 (that's just crazy!), B=5 (lipsticks dry out and develop bacteria and an unpleasant fragrance if they're too old), C=10

20. A=2, B=0, C=10

continued

21. A=10, B=2, C=10, D=0

22. A=0, B=10, C=0

23. A=4, B=6, C=-6, D=10

24. A=0, B=0, C=10

25. A=10, B=2, C=2, D=0

26. A=10, B=0, C=10, D=0

27. A=0, B=2, C=10

28. A=3, B=2 (*Every* day?), C=0, D=10

29. A=10, B=0 (*You'll damage it!*), C=4, D=6

30. A=0, B=8, C=10

ANALYSIS

Did you score from 280 to 306?

Congratulations! If you answered the questions in this self-assessment candidly, you have only moderate work to do on yourself—physically that is.

Your self-presentation is confident, and although I don't know you, I'd bet my bottom dollar you make a terrific impression on others. Although none of these answers is written in stone, it's your attitude about looking good that shows through here. You understand that you don't have to be born with perfect features in order to put your best face forward. You don't have to own a perfect body to walk in the world with beauty and confidence. You shop with smarts, you exercise regularly, and instead of eating everything that fits in your mouth, you eat only what you really want and need, rather than what they pile on your plate in restaurants. Most of all, you know that health comes first.

You're an individual; you're confident in your appearance; you attract the kind of people you want to hang with. Right?

See what tips you can pick up in the following chapter that will even further enhance the way you look and feel.

Did you score from 250 to 278?

You surely know how you'd like to look, but somehow you're not quite getting it all together.

This score indicates a woman who'd like to have a sense of style that's individual, but somehow she seems to follow fashion trends instead of developing her own best look. She's either too heavy or too thin—not at the weight that makes her feel most herself, most comfortable and pretty. She doesn't really know how to shop, doesn't know how to judge what's chic and what's tacky, even though she admires a "good" look on other women. She spends far too much money on her clothes and her makeup, and she knows it.

What's more, she'd like to occasionally offer some surprises in her look rather than being the same-old, same-old pretty-but-predictable self, but she doesn't know where to start. Most of the time her appearance makes her feel reasonably good, but she doesn't feel she has a true beauty "identity."

Is this you? Read on, sister.

Did you score from 200 to 248?

You are definitely not your most gorgeous.

You may not have changed your look since you were eighteen—not because you were so satisfied with the eighteen-year-old you, but because you simply don't know where to start. You love to see the models and the stars shining in the magazines, but how in the world can you adapt their look to yours if you're heavier, shorter, poorer? Read on!

Your old beauty goals are simply not appropriate anymore now that you're all grown up and out in the real world. Although they work reasonably well, your clothes no longer feel "friendly" to you—that is, you somehow don't feel as comfortable, attractive, and happy in them as you did some years ago.

Perhaps you need to reconstitute your look—your face, body, hair, and makeup—to fit the interesting woman you've become, but the woman nobody can see when they first meet you.

Before you can love yourself, before anyone can find the real you to love, you need to look more like the women you admire—and that is definitely within your power. I hope my own story that follows, and my own solutions, will guide you to self-love, then to the love of your life.

Did you score under 200?

Honey, I want to help you. This isn't a terrific score—and you know it.

This is why you're not physically prepared to meet the man of your dreams: you don't feel as well, as pretty, and as stylish as you should.

First of all, you often confuse cash with class, but all the expensive products in the world won't bring you an appearance that's filled with panache, dazzle, and imagination.

continued

Second of all, for all intents and purposes, you've stopped paying attention to your weight, your clothes, your makeup, and your hair because it just seems too daunting a task, right?

Finally—and this is the most serious—you probably can't walk as fast as you should, climb hills with as much energy, or even stay up as late as you used to. The fact is, your physical body is not at its prime—it slows you down, Kendra—I know it!

Don't settle for mediocre and ordinary: be the best you can be! Let today, the day you picked up this book, be the first day of the rest of your life, the best of your life.

I did it—and I was even too tired to shop before I decided to reconstitute my physical self. That was pretty serious. If I can help you, I'll be the happiest sister in the world.

❋   ❋   ❋

Lookin' Good

So, this chapter is about lookin' good. I've heard some people say that only frivolous, shallow people care that much about how they look. I think that frivolous, shallow people are the ones who *don't* care about how they look. More serious, deeper people are smart enough to know better. So, who should care about appearances?

You should care.

For starters, throughout history and cross-sections of various cultures, women have transformed their appearances and used their hair, makeup, and clothing to conform to a beauty ideal. There must be some inherent reason for this—can zillions of women be crazy? Not likely. Fact is, you can find scientific study after study informing us that today attractively turned-out people have a much better chance of getting hired, getting promoted, and landing clients and fat paychecks.

Like it or not, attractive women also attract more exciting men—and I'm not talking drop-dead, naturally beautiful, movie-star women: I'm talking women who know a little something about fashion and makeup. I'm talking women who have learned how to package their product—themselves. Good-looking people have a better shot at being noticed in a positive way than people who are sloppy about appearances. And although I wouldn't go so far as to endorse Billy Crystal's Fernando character on *Saturday Night Live,* who says, "You look mahvelous—it's better to look good than to feel good," he's not altogether crazy. It is important to always feel good, and looking good is an ingredient to feeling good. And, as we say in Brooklyn, "not for nuthin'," say what you like, people do judge others by their appearances. And here's one for Fernando: when you know you look good, you feel good. Tell me that's not so.

Some General Rules

I think I resent more than anything, now that I've lost some weight, when people say to me, "Oh my God, you look so good." Once I asked my husband, "Al, did I look so horrible before?" and he answered, "No, baby, you just looked different, but now I think you look happier, which makes you look better."

So, that's **rule number one.** When you pull yourself together, feel happier, and look better to yourself—you look better to everyone else. When I'm dressed in my favorite dress and I put on a pair of good shoes that I got on sale for $19.95, and some woman (forget about the guys) says to me, "Oooooh, those are the greatest shoes," few things make me happier. My self-esteem soars to a million.

Rule number two? Think of yourself as a package: you know when you give a gift, the wrapping counts as much as the present. It will take a while for Mr. Right to find out what a doll lives inside the package, but in order to attract his interest, the outside wrapping has to be sweet.

Rule number three? Pulling yourself together doesn't mean only when you have a big date or going to your cousin's wedding. I don't want to put pressure on you, sister, but I think you should try to look your best whenever you leave the house, and, if you have a good-looking neighbor who may want to borrow a cup of sugar, even when you're *in* your own house. When you walk your dog or run out for a quart of OJ, feel good about how you look: your future might be waiting at the counter in the corner deli. If you don't feel great about your appearance, you won't look him in the eye and do all the little come-on tricks that are a prelude to saying hello. He'll drive off into the sunset, and you'll drive off a cliff in disappointment. Personally speaking, I'm a glamour girl 24/7. You will never see me outside without my fake lashes. If you're my friend, and I'm lying in a hospital bed so sick I don't even know who's around me, please have somebody assigned to come in every day and glue on those eyelashes. If you want me to get better, don't let me lie there without the lashes—oh God, I'll know it from somewhere deep within, and it will make me crazy and very insecure, and I'll lose my will to live. I'll take the real mink lashes, please, as opposed to the synthetic mink. No, wait, maybe paste on the purple ones—I'll need a laugh.

Rule number four? This chapter will mainly cover the rudiments of fashion, makeup, and hair as I practice them, but if you want to be your most gorgeous, be aware of the other packaging ploys:

* Visit your dentist. There's nothing as pretty as a white-toothed smile, and today there are inexpensive ways of getting those teeth gorgeous—even if you took a gray-tooth-making antibiotic when you were little.
* Check your breath—either by having your very good friend smell when you exhale, or blow into a small paper bag and smell what comes out.
* Smoking is pretty horrible both for your health and certainly for your teeth and breath.
* A boozy breath is the worst.
* Get manicures and pedicures. If you bite your nails, this is the one perfect way to encourage yourself to stop.
* Finally, do I have to say this—do you look clean? Do you have a nail brush to get the grime out? Is your hair oily and limp-hanging? Are the pores in the oily places on your face speckled with blackheads? *Arrrrrgh.*

But I bet you clean up good. Do it.

Fashion

*Put even the plainest woman into a beautiful dress,
and unconsciously she will try to live up to it.*

LUCILE, LADY DUFF-GORDON

Only God helps the badly dressed.

SPANISH PROVERB

I have always felt that fashion is a cool form of self-expression available to anyone, no matter how rich or poor. Dressing up has always been my favorite game since I was very small, and here's the way I play it.

Suppose you feel mousy or awkward. Suppose you really don't know where to start being fashion savvy? Here's an idea: be someone else.

If I'm not feeling particularly Star-like when I'm out buying a new outfit, I'll often think, "Who *doesn't* feel mousy today? I'll bet Halle Berry doesn't feel mousy." Then, I'll project—I'll be Halle for a couple of hours, I'll try to take on her mind-set and look at clothes in the stores through her eyes. Now, I don't mean you or I ought to dress exactly like Halle if one of us has a size 16 butt, but only try to emulate her confidence and know-how. Becoming Halle once in a while allows me to go out there and serve it up.

Here's my fashion philosophy: you become a new person every time you put on a new outfit. Last week when I went to the tennis match, I was definitely the black Audrey Hepburn. I had on the black picture hat, the little purse, the delicately flowered dress. Never mind that she was a size 2. I was Audrey, kids. Here's another thing: I never mind looking different from what others expect from Star because I know who I really am. That translates into if I wake up in a Sheryl Crow jeans state of mind, I'm not intimidated by someone who woke up in an Audrey Hepburn state of mind.

The truth is that clothes allow me to be someone unique every day and to have fun at it. Fashion is fun; I don't do very much in life anymore that doesn't bring me joy and happy up my outlook.

If a bad hair day can change your whole outlook for that day, a bad outfit can do the same thing. I believe this: the way people look at you, the way you march through your life depends heavily on how attractively you're turned out. You may be the wisest, finest potential friend or lover in the world, but few people get to the inside of you until they check out the outside. Your appearance has to be appealing—and that's the truth. You can't judge a book by its cover, true, but a great cover sure entices you to the read.

When I was ready to look for the man who would be my life's companion—or rather, when I was ready for him to look for me—I also started to pay greater attention to my clothes. This wasn't exactly the hardest task ahead of me, because when it comes to fashion, I'm a willing girl. Still, in my life, so far, I've always had two impediments to looking like what every magazine told me was attractive. The first impediment was money—or lack of it. When I was young, I was thin, but I didn't have money to buy the good clothes I admired. When I was older, I had the money, but then I also had the excess weight. High-class fashion designers, the original thinkers who dress the magazine models, definitely were not designing for me.

So, I always had to be creative within the context of my own needs. The first thing I did creatively was develop my most sacred fashion mantra.

Thou Shall Not Pay Retail

There is almost nothing that you love in any magazine that can't be inexpensively duplicated. We're so lucky to live in a world where clothing outlets are ubiquitous and elegant bargains are everywhere—if only you know the location of the places where they hang. Some of my fabulous friends can buy Chanel direct from the Parisian shows, and although now I can afford to do the same, I choose not to. I love a great bargain. My personal motto is "You can fake it even when you make it." I love to put outfits together that look and feel expensive but are not. Included in this chapter is Star's Insider Guide to Fabulous Fashion Finds all across America and internationally too. But how do you know what's a fashion find, and how do you know if it's for you? Here are some basics where I suggest you start:

Cut Off Their Heads

For as many years as I can remember, I've clipped photographs of beautiful women wearing the clothes I thought I loved from the newest fashion magazines. Then I'd paste the photos on the inside of my closet door. Well, actually not the whole photo. I'd always decapitate the photos of the models or movie stars wearing the clothes (who annoyed me no end because I could *never* look or be like them). Say I saw a great photograph of Nicole Kidman wearing navy blue pants and a navy blue crewneck sweater with a cute Peter Pan collar blouse, I'd cut out the picture, minus Nicole's head, and hang the photo on the inside of my closet door. It would hang there for a couple of weeks while I studied the look, deciding if it would be good for me. Sometimes, I'd put a photo of my own face on a photograph in place of, say, Catherine Deneuve's. If Deneuve was wearing a little navy blue Chanel suit with the gold buttons and the delicate gold chain belt, I'd decide if it genuinely was a look that would be good for me.

Now, Kidman and Deneuve are both a whole lot more slender than I was, and very white and blonde to boot, but we did have one thing in common: I knew I could wear *classic* with style, and they were nothing if not classic. So, if the answer was yes to the look, I duplicated it. On the trail of Chanel, I'd go to Lane Bryant or a small boutique up in Harlem, buy the best navy blue suit I could find, go to a store that sells vintage buttons (there are many of them in every big city), and carefully sew original (or copies of) Chanel gold buttons on the suit jacket. Then, I'd find a gold chain belt as close to the Deneuve picture as possible. I'd find a fabulous copy of those long Chanel pearls. I'd emulate the look— and when I finished, I tell you, it would take a Chanel scholar to know I was faking it. Making it by faking it.

I have to be real here. When I weighed over 250 pounds and cut out a photo of Halle Berry wearing a body-skimming satin dress, I had to live in the truth of what I was and what my body was. As true as the fact that I couldn't afford real Chanel back in that day, I also couldn't dress like Halle Berry. Her dress would not work for me—for my butt, for my breasts, for my waist. Big deal. There were plenty of other role models.

The best thing you can do for yourself is to cut out photographs of those who have body types similar to yours, from the start: it makes life easier. If you can't bring yourself to cut off their heads, draw little mustaches on them so you aren't intimidated by their perfection.

You have to assume that those people in *Vogue* and *Harper's Bazaar* have plenty of money to spend, so steal their expertise! And when you wear the duplication, strut your stuff, baby. Diva everyone with your attitude. Don't be meek, don't wait for tables in crowded restaurants, don't take no for an answer when you're negotiating.

Educate Yourself

No one is born knowing what "good" looks like. You have to observe and hang out with people who shop well, then use them as mentors to learn what quality fashion looks like. Browsing the great department or specialty stores also is an education. Go into a fine leather store in the closest big city. Touch a leather coat or purse to feel how soft and supple it is. Check out the lining in an Amsale gown; see how it's sewn with the tiniest of hand stitches and attached to the gown. Then check out a leather purse or coat in a low-quality/low-price store: see how the latter feels brittle and crackly in your hand. See how linings are either glued on or sewn with careless machine stitches.

Just as an example, let me decode the inspection of a good leather purse.

First, touch the leather of the purse. Does it feel like *buttah,* soft, delicious? Good. Open up the bag. Does it have a fabric or suede interior? If it's suede, is it real or synthetic? Does the purse have several compartments for you to safely store your valuables? Check the zippers in the interior compartments—do they stick or move smoothly up and down? See how the zipper is finished off: it's best if there's some sort of leather jacket covering the zipper edges. Check the purse straps—how are they attached to the body of the purse? The straps on really good pocketbooks are stitched onto the body of the bag, not just held to the bag by a grommet.

Then I personally evaluate how I'm going to carry the bag. If it's a clutch, I stand holding it in my hand the way I'm going to carry it, and check out my reflection in the mirror. Do I like the way it looks in my hand? I walk around with the bag. If it's a clutch and it feels too big in your hand when you walk around the store, it's sure going to feel too big at a cocktail party. If it's a shoulder bag and doesn't hang smoothly, lightly, and securely on your shoulder, it'll drive you crazy when you get it home. If you're a student carrying books, a parent grabbing for your kids, or a list maker always jotting something down, you need a shoulder bag, not a clutch purse. When you shop, everyone *definitely* needs a shoulder bag: there's never anyplace to put your clutch when you're frantically going through the racks.

One more thing: I know what I always need to carry with me, no matter what the occasion. Every woman knows what her essentials consist of—keys, cell phone, lipstick, powder, maybe a PDA? Reading glasses? Contact lens solution? Maybe just two of those things. It's different for everybody. When I'm out handbag shopping, I always put these essentials in a small, self-sealing plastic storage bag (so nothing soils the prospective purse), and before I decide to buy, I see if the bag fits in the purse. I never buy a handbag that won't fit my needs.

Knowing Real vs. Getting a Steal

So, now you've educated yourself as to what "good" feels like. But perhaps "good" is too expensive. Your education is not wasted: now you've got to look for a purse that's similar but inexpensive. Here's a hint: buy the fashion magazines that do the comparison thing—you know, splurge vs. steal, real vs. faux, dream vs. bargain. They always come out at the top of the season when fall or spring merchandise will soon be released. Now rip out the handbag page, the shoe page, the accessory page: these are your cheat sheets—they'll help you decide on which faux is closest to the real. If the hottest new bag is a Gucci purse with enamel snakes on it, you know you can't really duplicate that Gucci purse, but you know that leather with some sort of enamel ornamentation is the style this season.

Where will you find the less expensive version? I note that within about three weeks that the real designer purse (or shoes or accessories or jewelry or whatever you're searching for) comes out, the less expensive interpretation becomes available in the department stores and fabulous stores like Payless Shoe Source.

Also, check my Insider Guide, below. If you find yourself in Pisa, skip the Leaning Tower and go to an Armani outlet. If you're in Palm Beach, skip the beach and visit a jewelry outlet and pick up a little Bulgari-look necklace for $300—the original is $30,000. Oh my God, I can't stand it!

The One Always-Works Outfit

Find one. Let it be the outfit that makes you feel most adorable or sexy or persuasive. Have two hanging in your closet.

For me, at any size, it's the little black dress. Because I like my arms, it's usually sleeveless. I like a simple round collar and a hem length that hits me at the knees. I can wear it with long pearls, with short pearls, with a great gold chain. I can put on a jacket and make it perfect for work or evening—depending on the jacket.

It's interesting to think of clothes as costume. Wherever you go, whatever role you happen to be playing at the moment—job seeker? true-love seeker? party-goer?—your costume should be appropriate to the role. With a sharply tailored but simple jacket, that little black dress on me could address a jury anywhere. A magnificent brocade or velvet or satin jacket and that little black dress could take me to *The View* and out to dinner that evening. High heels dress it up, low heels dress it down. Today I have several little black dresses. But when I had no money, one black dress worked for every role. Job interview? Black dress, tailored jacket, pearls. First date at lunch? No necklace at all—just the V of my dress showing a bit of décolletage, sandals, and puh-lease—never, never pantyhose with sandals. (No matter if it's footless, toeless—you'll still look crazy if you wear open-toed sandals with pantyhose. Bad, bad.) Fancy-schmancy evening affair? Same black dress, only with a pretty evening shawl, my hair pulled up, and cheap *triple*-strand pearls. Do you know I still have the triple-strand pearls I bought twenty years ago for $18? Today, I mix them with the *real* pearls I got as a gift—and defy you to tell the difference by just looking.

Pants

Three rules on pants, girls.

1. No side pockets that stick out: those big old stupid side pockets add ten pounds before you turn around—especially if you have a well-endowed booty. Pockets must be flush with your body.
2. If you are trying to minimize your tummy, buy pants only with a flat front, side zip. All the really great designers—Armani, Calvin Klein, Ralph Lauren—use a side zip with a beautiful waistband, giving the sleekest look in town.
3. Must wear pleats? Not my favorite, but you can if you wear drop pleats that start at the hip, not pleats that start at the waist and end at the knee—okay? A pleat on the hip is going to widen and bulk you up, trust Aunt Star. Remember Seinfeld's puffy shirt? More than two pleats on pants gives you *puffy crotch*—not a great look.

A Few Words on Shoes

On this, I could write a whole book. I'll spare you. However, I believe that shoes are the windows to the soul (or sole . . . if you want to be cute). So, do this little exercise with me:

* Take out the three pairs of shoes that you (1) love, (2) wear the most, (3) wear when you really want to impress.
* Put them on the floor and ask yourself the following questions: Is the heel scratched? Is one side more worn or uneven? Is the buckle or bow or elastic scratched, broken, safety-pinned?
* If you answer yes to any of these questions, you may not wear those shoes again.

Here are the shoe rules:

✳ You may not wear shoes where the heels are scratched or that little tap thing on the bottom of the heel is abused. If the little tap thing is actually missing, you'll click when you walk. Don't do it. For three dollars, the shoemaker will put a new one on the bottom of your heel, so you won't click.

✳ Shoes have to be comfortable. Anytime anyone can look at you walking down the street and say to herself, "That girl's feet hurt," you're not in a good shoe. If they hurt in the shoe store when you try them on, they never get better.

✳ My favorite high-end shoes come from Giuseppie Zanotti, Gucci, Manolo Blahnik, Rene Caovilla, and Jimmy Choo. My favorite inexpensive shoes are, what else, Payless—I love their sandals, wedgies, and flip-flops, and my Starlet by Star Jones designs give you high-end glamour for $19.99.

✳ Never shop for shoes late in the day when your feet are swollen. Early in the morning is the best time.

✳ If you're someone who wears hose all the time, try on shoes with hose. But I don't want to hear about you wearing hose with open-toed sandals.

Does It *Have* to Match?

No. The last thing you want to be is too matchy-matchy. That even translates into a handbag and shoes—the traditional matched set. If the colors come from the same family, even if they don't match, the combination will be perfect— mauve and purple, gray and black, teal and blue look fine and even better than mauve and mauve or gray and gray. This does not include orange. I suggest losing the orange. If you *must* do, say, orange shoes, do a purse with a pattern in it that includes orange. For God's sakes, with the orange shoes and the patterned purse, do *not* wear an orange jumpsuit. Remember: colors are accessories as much as jewelry is; keep them in balance.

Build your outfit around the fashion touch you want to emphasize. If I feel like dressing trashy one day when I'm cavorting around town with my girlfriends, I may decide on a floral halter dress in greens, pinks, and dark blues. The dress is my focal point, that's my primary. If I choose green rhinestone and crystal shoes with gold heels, everyone will look at the shoes and miss the dress—and it'll also be *too* trashy. So I'll settle on plucking out one subdued color from the floral pattern—maybe plain green—and it'll be pretty, but it won't compete with my dress. You define what you want to be primary—your new strappy shoes, a new necklace, a brooch? Everything else should enhance and show it off—not do battle with it.

Foundation Is All

No matter who you are, what size body you have, or what you look like, always wear a good foundation under your fashion choices. Choose the good bra that lifts you up, a thong with a little tummy support or Spanx (or a similar support garment) to hold in your hips (they're kind of like boy shorts or support panty-hose without the stockings). I don't know anyone who doesn't wear some sort of foundation.

What Not to Wear

Recently, a popular program called *What Not to Wear* hit our TV screens. It's popular because it's so negative and so true that it hits a nerve. Everyone should dress appropriately. For example, you wouldn't wear a super-low-cut dress to a funeral or shining satin pants to a Little League game. You wouldn't wear a backpack, headphones around your neck, a miniskirt that doesn't clear your thighs, or heavy makeup to a job interview (facial piercing, especially tongue jewelry, or visible tattoos are definitely a no-no unless you're interviewing for something *very* other than a Fortune 500 company). Don't carry a leather purse to an animal rights meeting, and don't wear clothes that don't fit anywhere, even to your mom's Thanksgiving dinner: spring for the extra few dollars to have your off-the-rack find tailored so it really is a find.

Bottom line: if you're not sure if something is appropriate, I'll bet anything you're sure of what's *not* appropriate. Don't wear it.

Controversial Fashion

Don't be intimidated by those who disagree with your choices. For example, I get blasted by a certain group because I wear fur. That's my choice. That's the greatest part of being an American—you get to have choices. Don't insist that I embrace the cause that's true to you. I will die for your right to go out and protest and express your opinion, but you may not attack me physically or try to intimidate me into believing what you believe. You've every right to express your opinion, and I've every right to reject it.

You know, I've seen members of a group attack me and others for wearing fur, while stepping over a homeless person without giving him a moment's thought—let alone a buck.

So, I will not insist you come down with me to deliver food to homebound AIDS patients with God's Love We Deliver, and don't you dare throw paint at me for wearing a fur coat or trust me; we're going to have a problem. Don't let this "chic chic foo foo" style thing fool you. I was raised in the Miller Homes housing projects and I don't play.

Red Carpet Glamazons

Thousands of years ago, in Asia Minor, women warriors called Amazons ruled the battlefield. They wielded spear and sword in defense of their children and motherland. The traditional image of the warrior Amazon woman was noble, courageous, intelligent, and above all, independent. The Amazons led their female armies into battle, they beat the guy warriors in archery and—a little known fact—they wore stunning tunics. The whole world bowed at their feet and tried to emulate their style. Did they walk on red carpets? Probably, at the victory balls.

Today, we have very few Amazons. What we have are Glamazons. These women are the most powerful and beautiful in all of Hollywood. The whole world bows at their feet. We try to emulate their style.

I'm an expert on Glamazons, and if you tuned in on Hollywood's Oscar night, you might have caught me interviewing some of them.

Here's my list of the ten most powerful Glamazons in Hollywood in their most shining moments. They rarely make a fashion faux pas. They've figured out what works on their bodies, and they stick with it. The true fashion Glamazons have definite style.

Star	Her Style	All-Star's Favorite Fashion
Nicole Kidman	**Sheer elegance**	**Black sheer Gaultier (2003 Oscars)**
Halle Berry	**Silver-screen goddess**	**Floral and burgundy Elie Saab (2001 Oscars)**
Jennifer Lopez	**Flair for the fabulous**	**Sea-foam green Valentino (2001 Oscars)**
Hilary Swank	**Long, lean, and luscious**	**Navy Guy Laroche (2005 Oscars)**
Jennifer Garner	**Always a lady**	**Coral Valentino (2004 Oscars)**
Penélope Cruz	**Sexy and chic**	**Givenchy blue chiffon (2005 Cannes Film Festival)**
Beyoncé	**Glamour and glitz**	**Atelier Versace's black silk velvet strapless "Siren" gown (2005 Oscars)**
Oprah Winfrey	**Classic glamour**	**Red Vera Wang (2005 Legends Ball)**
Charlize Theron	**Classic Hollywood**	**Blue John Galliano (2005 Oscars)**
Salma Hayek	**Va-va-va-voom**	**Blue Prada (2005 Oscars)**

Everything a Diva Needs to Know
to Rule the Red Carpet List

I got to see these Glamazons up close and personal as the red carpet host for E! Entertainment Television's Academy Awards night specials in 2005, and, sure, they have the bodies and the designer clothes, but they also have some tricks that make everything work! Of course, I wanted to know how it is done, so I asked Julie Alderfer, my longtime wardrobe mistress at *The View* to give me the wardrobe tricks of the trade.

Quick Fixes
To Common Problems That Occur on the
Red Carpet . . . or On the Way to Meet Your In-laws

Problem No. 1: Jiggling or Sagging Breast
Solution: A strapless, supportive bra that fits snugly around the ribs and is ample in the cup size to insert pads underneath (foam inserts or shoulder pads work) for lift and cleavage (www.bratenders.com). Or, depending on the cut of the gown, *Braza* makes adhesive tape to place over the breast area, a temporary lift (www.brazabra.com).

Problem No. 2: Nipple Showing through Blouse
Solution: *Braza* makes an adhesive-backed bra in light, medium, and dark. Choose your color and cup size. Cut out areola-size circles and press on nipples. Make sure to press out the wrinkles on the tape and flatten your nipple bump at the same time. (This takes expertise, so cut out several for practice.) (www.brazabra.com or www.bratenders.com) *Angel's Secret* are silicone nipple covers with a special adhesive inside. They can be worn repeatedly (www.laurensilva.com or www.manhattanwardrobesupply.com).

Problem No. 3: Tummy Looks "Poochy"

Solution: The lower the dress is cut in back, the greater the challenge because the support garment may show. *Spanx* makes an excellent tummy tucker, but better choose a dress that's cut higher in the back, or hold your stomach in (www.spanx.com).

Problem No. 4: You Have Schmutz on Your Dress

Solution: Baby wipes are a wardrobe-kit essential. They are the best for removing makeup as well as dirt of all origins. Remember to dab (don't rub in the stain) and turn the wipe as you dab. Be sure to buy the unscented wipes. *Janie* spot cleaner works well on grease stains. Rub on and brush off with the built-in brush. Repeat until the spot disappears. Try white wine on a red-wine stain. My favorite stain remover is *Zout* (www.manhattanwardrobesupply.com or your local hardware or variety store).

Problem No. 5: You Shaved Too Quickly and Got Nicked

Solution: Do it the old-fashioned way and stick pieces of cigarette paper on the nick until the bleeding stops. Or use L'Occitane's Cade shaving stick—it has potassium alum, which is a great astringent.

Problem No. 6: You Got Your Period and There Is a Spot on Your White Pants

Solution: The enzymes in your saliva will get out your stain. A little spit on a clean cloth or a baby wipe, dab, then rinse with cold water—and it's gone.

Problem No. 7: Your Bra Strap Breaks

Solution: Tiny black lingerie pins are essential for emergencies. They have a dull finish, and they hide and hold. They can be found at www.manhattanwardrobe-supply.com or the sewing department of your local variety store.

Problem No. 8: Your Hem Rips

Solution: If you're near an iron and can't sew, have *Stitchwitchery* on hand. It is sold in rolls. Insert a ½"-wide strip between hem layers and carefully press with an iron. It sticks like glue, so don't iron directly on the product. Can be found at

continued

www.manhattanwardrobesupply.com. Vapon's *Topstick* is an essential in your wardrobe kit. It is double-stick tape that adheres to skin and fabric. Great for hems. Can be found at Sally Beauty Supply Stores. Can be found locally, nation-wide, and at www.sallybeauty.com.

Problem No. 9: There Are Sweat Stains on the Underarms of Your Dress
Solution: Scented deodorant discolors the underarms of your clothing. Switch to unscented antiperspirant for the red carpet. *Zout* helps with the stain or dab some hydrogen peroxide on the area. Rinse well. Adhesive-backed disposable dress shields can be cut to fit your gown. No sweat.

Star Awards

Admit it. There are some women who make you want to jump up and down when you see them, make you want to yell, "Bravo, girl!" You're not jealous, nor are you a "hater" with these girls. You don't even react in that way we sometimes do when we feel threatened—you just have to admit that the sister has it going on. Here are the women who I think definitely have it going on. You have your list—this is mine:

Star's Fabulous Six . . . Just Because They Are

Best Avant Garde Princess	**Gwen Stefani**
Best Trendsetter	**Jennifer Lopez**
Best Legendary Divas	**Barbara Walters and Nancy Wilson**
Best Sexy Siren	**Angelina Jolie**
Best Dressed, Period	**Halle Berry**

Even Cheaper, Even Chicer

* **Visit the vintage stores.** Certain clothes just seem to assume that a beautiful and fascinating woman will be wearing them. Ironically, they're often found in dusty vintage clothing shops, and although they come from the nineteen twenties, thirties, forties, and fifties, they're timeless. You can mix antique looks with trendy styles and emerge with extraordinary style. I bought a blue beaded top in such a vintage store that Diana Vreeland might have worn, and then found brand-new and exactly matching St. John pants. A Balenciaga ball gown or a Fortuny velvet jacket can be bought for a fraction of what it cost new—even fifty years ago! A forties man's antique satin cummerbund can dress up a new wool shift. This look is for the original and the daring who appreciate the finest fashion.

* **Visit the auction houses.** Every large city and small town has an auction house. Ask when they'll be selling "old clothes," and make time for a browse. The most interesting items can be inexpensively purchased at such auctions. An exquisite lace Victorian nightgown can be altered by a dressmaker to create the most beautiful summer party dress. Beaded bags, embroidered jackets—let your creativity roam wild.

* **Visit your little corner dressmaker.** Have a dress/skirt/suit you love and wish you'd bought two of twenty years ago? A good dressmaker can duplicate it or, as a matter of fact, copy anything you bring to her. A photograph of a Chanel suit in this month's *Vogue* can be copied and whipped up for a fraction of the cost Coco would have charged.

* **Visit the good department stores at sale time.** Ask the information lady in any fine department store when the yearly sale will occur, and plan to spend the morning shopping. Sales often occur after Christmas and in mid-August. Real bargains are available here, and because the merchandise is top-notch, you do better than in a tacky store that sports cheaper (in every way) goods, all year long.

* **Visit the showrooms.** Some major fashion designers open their

showrooms to the public once or twice a year as a goodwill gesture or perhaps to sell slightly model-worn merchandise. Call the offices of your favorite designers (Armani? Bill Blass? Yves Saint Laurent?) and ask if the public is ever permitted to browse and buy. Unfortunately, this happens only in major cities: you won't find a Givenchy showroom in HoHoKus, New Jersey.

✦ **Visit the street.** If you live in a big city, you're familiar with the street vendors who sell the inexpensive copies (or interpretations, as I like to call them) of the costlier versions. Sure, it's not nice and, in some cases, probably illegal to rip off the name brands, but it's not breaking a law to buy them—in fact, I think that occasional shopping at the vendors on the block is the quintessential definition of street smarts. If you know what the real thing looks like (and do your homework here—go to the good department stores to closely inspect the product that's being emulated), sometimes you can find an interpretation that's almost indistinguishable from the original. It's one-millionth the price. Purses, jewelry, watches—even some beautiful clothes are readily available on a vendor's makeshift metal table. Think about it.

What Goes On in the Discount Stores, Stays in the Discount Stores

Where is it written that you have to pay full price for looking good? The savviest women I know, even the wealthiest women I know are drawn by the scent of a bargain. Don't get in their way; don't get in my way when Prada beckons at a discounted price.

Okay: Here it is, my Insider Guide to Fabulous Fashion Finds. But don't tell everybody, please. I'm about to break my own rule and hip everyone to my favorite places to shop cheaply, but it's a good idea in general not to give all your secrets away. If you find a really, really, really good outlet that sells really, really, really good "interpretations" of Versace suits, and if you tell all your acquaintances, everyone will have your look. Not great. That's one of the reasons, in all honesty, I like to shop alone.

Here are my true confessions: I used to shop alone because I was a bigger girl than my girlfriends. It wasn't that I was uncomfortable watching them pull on the teeny-tiny jeans that wouldn't fit on my thigh. I was uncomfortable because I was selfish. I didn't want to sit around watching you put on size 6 jeans when I needed to get to Lane Bryant for my size 18. But now that I'm thinner, I still feel the same way. When I'm shopping, I'm shopping for me, not for you, and I don't have that much time these days for that pleasure. I could have been done and gone to the next location while you were just taking off your third pair of something. I know what looks good on me, I know what I like, and I don't *need* even good friends telling me how fabulous or unfabulous something is. Now, if you're one of my girls and you need to shop for something special and you want me to come along for support and advice, I'm there, with my whole heart. But that's not shopping for me. That I do alone at my special places.

Now that I'm making it all public, I'll see you at the secret places, girl! Don't get too chatty—I'm there to get things done.

Star's Insider Guide to Fabulous Fashion Finds

I don't know why anyone would pay full price for an Escada dress, a Chanel suit, an Armani coat, a Loro Piana cashmere throw, a Carolina Herrera wedding dress, Ferragamo shoes, or a Bottega Veneta purse when you can buy these and hundreds of thousands of other items at discounts from 15 to up to 75 percent at the designer outlets. Don't be intimidated by the names of these fancy stores—remember, we're stepping up our look here. The fashion magazines tell us what is hot; we're just getting what's hot at a cool price.

While there have always been smaller discount stores in most communities that carried nice quality and brand-name merchandise at greatly reduced prices (Loehmann's, TJ Maxx, Bolton's, Target, or Burlington Coat Factory, for example), you're lucky to be living in a decade where the art of the fabulous fashion find has been taken to new heights. I've traveled to those heights, and I tell you, there are fashion treasures to be found up there at incredibly low prices.

Mark It Down and They Will Come

The really exciting finds are usually unearthed in places called outlet or factory centers, and each has its own merchants who rent space from the center. Most are to be found on the Internet under "Shopping Outlet Centers," and many have stores from coast to coast.

Basic Internet Research 101

1. Log onto the Internet (via AOL or Internet Explorer, etc.)
2. Type in the search engine Web address. Good ones I use are:
   - www.google.com
   - www.yahoo.com
   - www.askjeeves.com
3. Type in specifics of what you are looking for in the search box:
   - If you want a particular location try: "Shopping Outlet Center Michigan"
   - If you want a particular store in a particular location try: "Shopping Outlet Center Chanel Michigan"

Make no mistake: this is not ordinary mall shopping. The outlets are designed for upscale, fashion-conscious shoppers who are looking for top-quality and designer labels. Still, every outlet is not the same as every other because some offer a far larger selection of the highest-quality merchandise, and some offer more of the midline stores like the Gap, Old Navy, Jones of New York, and Nike.

The marvelous thing about all this is that no matter where you live in the United States and in many areas where you might be traveling in Europe, Japan, or Mexico—or in a million other places—you can probably find an outlet center not far from where you are. Many of these outlets can be found together online, if you plug "fashion outlet centers" into your search engine.

And here's a great tip: most of these outlets have deals with bus and limousine companies to ferry passengers from a spot close to their homes to the center of the outlet. Just call or e-mail the outlet that sounds most terrific and ask for its public transportation schedules.

In addition to individual outlet centers composed of thousands of specialty stores selling their own top brand merchandise (like Coach, Celine, Loro Piana, Judith Lieber, Gucci, Ralph Lauren, Kenneth Cole, Seiko watches, Godiva chocolate, Crabtree & Evelyn, Dress Barn, Waterford crystal, Betsey Johnson, Etro, and Armani, for example), many fine department stores have their own outlet stores within the larger outlet center. There they sell their merchandise at vastly reduced rates because it may be last season's or this season's unsold but perfect merchandise. Saks Fifth Avenue, for example, has stores called Off 5th in outlets all over the country. Barneys and Brooks Brothers and many other great department stores all operate factory outlets, and the bargains to be found there are amazing.

Here's a bonus feature very few people know about, even those who customarily frequent designer outlets: if you go to the Web site of the particular outlet, and click on Coupons or Sales and Events, you'll often be able to print out an extra certificate for approximately 15–25 percent off your already bargain-priced purchases. Some outlets require that you join a "shopper's club," which is usually free and consists of just giving them your name and address online to get the discount coupons and coupon books. **Star tip:** use a fake e-mail address so you don't have to give out yours. My favorite catch e-mail site is www.dodgeit.com. You can make up an e-mail address (*lovestoshop@discount .com*, for example) and go there to check it. All you have to do is look up the name you used and any mail you've received is right there, and it doesn't clutter up your real e-mail address. Plus it's free. Use it girl!

A point to remember: if you're searching for a particular brand or designer, the Internet can again be enormously helpful. On the Web, call up the outlet that you suspect might carry your dream shoes, type in the designer or brand name, and you'll immediately see if the center near you offers those particular beauties.

Okay: here is the information you crave—and most of these outlets have locations coast to coast.

Star's Guide to the Best Outlet Shopping in America

✳ *Chicago Premium Outlets*

1650 Premium Outlets Boulevard
Aurora, IL 60502
(630) 585-2200
www.premiumoutlets.com/chicago
Mon–Sat 10–9, Sun 10–6
Brands: 120 stores, including Adidas, BCBG Max Azria, Elie Tahari, MaxMara, Miss Sixty, Salvatore Ferragamo, Theory, and Versace.
Star tips: Go for the high-end stuff—you can get the best deals.

✳ *The Crossings Premium Outlets*

1000 Route 611
Tannersville, PA 18372
(570) 629-4650
www.premiumoutlets.com/thecrossings
Mon–Sat 10–9, Sun 10–6
Brands: 100 stores, including Ann Taylor, Burberry, Calvin Klein, Coach, DKNY Jeans, Ellen Tracy, and Polo Ralph Lauren.
Star tips: This is just basic—find out when the sales are.

✳ *Desert Hills Premium Outlets*

48400 Seminole Drive
Cabazon, CA 92230
(951) 849-6641
www.premiumoutlets.com/deserthills
Sun–Thu 10–8, Fri 10–9, Sat 9–9

Brands: 130 stores, including A/X Armani Exchange, Barneys New York, BCBG Max Azria, Christian Dior, Dolce & Gabbana, Gucci, Juicy Couture, Lacoste, Miu Miu, Prada, TSE, and Yves Saint Laurent Rive Gauche.

Star tips: This outlet has rightly been called "a desert oasis." It's about an hour east of Los Angeles but worth the trip. The best deals can be found at BCBG and Burberry. I spent three hours in Gucci once 7 years ago and found shoes (that I still own and wear) that were originally $600 and I got them for $99!!! OK . . . so I bought four pairs, but who's counting?

✳ *Great Lakes Crossing*

4000 Baldwin Road
Auburn Hills, MI 48326
(248) 454-5010
(877) SHOP-GLC
www.shopgreatlakescrossing.com
Mon–Sat 10–9, Sun 11–6

Brands: 200 stores, including Bose, Frederick's of Hollywood, Max Studio, Neiman Marcus Last Call, Off 5th Saks Fifth Avenue, TJ Maxx, and Victoria's Secret.

Star tips: Shopping till you drop is actually a possibility at this 1.4-million-square-foot mall. The best deals are on the clearance racks carrying clothes from last season where you can find clothes up to 70 percent off.

✳ *Leesburg Corner Premium Outlets*

241 Fort Evans Road NE
Leesburg, VA 20176
(703) 737-3071
www.premiumoutlets.com/leesburg
Mon–Sat 10–9, Sun 11–6
Brands: 110 stores, including Burberry, Calvin Klein, Kenneth Cole, Off 5th Saks Fifth Avenue, and Polo Ralph Lauren.
Star tips: The best shops here are Burberry and Off 5th, where you can find beautiful clothing for half off. Go straight to the designer section of Off 5th—that's where the real finds are.

✳ *Loehmann's*

Locations nationwide, check Web site for a specific location
www.loehmanns.com
Loehmann's is not an outlet but an individual fashion discount store with fifty branches coast to coast. Trust me—it's absolutely wonderful. I start at the Back Room in every Loehmann's store I visit for the most exciting designer names. You can find Armani, Gucci, and all the good stuff.

✳ *Orlando Premium Outlets*

8200 Vineland Avenue
Orlando, FL 32821
(407) 238-7787
www.premiumoutlets.com/orlando
Mon–Sat 10–10, Sun 10–9
Brands: 110 stores, including Anne Klein, Burberry, Fendi, Giorgio Armani, Kenneth Cole, Salvatore Ferragamo, Theory, and Versace.
Star tips: The quality of this outlet is superb. It carries some of the finest designer labels and has a great selection of sizes and styles. Leave the kids at Disney World and go find your version of the "Happiest Place on Earth."

✳ *Prime Outlets San Marcos*

3939 IH-35 South #900
San Marcos, TX 78666
(800) 628-9465
www.primeoutlets.com
Mon–Sat 10–9, Sun 11–6
Brands: Adrienne Vittadini, Coach, Cole Haan, Dooney & Bourke, Furla, Neiman Marcus Last Call, Off 5th Saks Fifth Avenue, Polo Ralph Lauren, and Tumi.
Star tips: You'll have to do some searching, but you can find great deals here, especially on Dooney & Bourke handbags.

✳ *The Secaucus Outlets*

20 Enterprise Avenue North
Secaucus, NJ 07094
(201) 348-4780
www.harmonmeadow.com
Mon, Tue, Wed 10–6; Thurs 10–8;
Fri, Sat 10–7; Sun 11–6
Brands: Over 100 stores, including Century 21, Jil Sander, Tahari, Tommy Hilfiger, and Yves Saint Laurent.
Star tips: Century 21 is a great store for finding wonderful designer pieces. You can find Lagerfeld winter coats for a fraction of their retail prices. Century 21 also has a store in New York City.

✳ *Tanger Outlet Centers*

1770 West Main Street
Riverhead, NY 11901
(800) 407-4894
www.tangeroutlet.com
Mon–Sat 9–9, Sun 10–8

Brands: 168 stores, including ABC Carpet & Home, Barneys New York, Coach, Calvin Klein, Kenneth Cole, Polo Ralph Lauren, and Tumi.
Star tips: There are multiple locations nationwide. Log onto their Web site for the location closest to you. In the summer, I make several trips here.

❖ *Woodbury Common Premium Outlets*

498 Red Apple Court
Central Valley, NY 10917
(845) 928-4000
www.premiumoutlets.com/woodburycommon
Daily 10–9
Brands: 220 stores, including Celine, Dolce & Gabbana, Escada, Fendi, Giorgio Armani, Gucci, Tod's, and Versace.
Star tips: The best of the best! This is my favorite outlet in the country. I've found $4,000 Armani evening dresses here for $169! Don't go into St. John because I have already bought everything in my size that is on sale!

Okay, now remember . . .

Outlet Rules

1. If the item you purchase is on sale, ask to make sure it's returnable. Most outlets set their own rules, and often, clearance items are not returnable.
2. Many outlets will allow you to return stuff in any of their outlet stores. Ask.
3. Most outlets will *not* let you return merchandise to their non-outlet stores. Don't expect to buy shoes at Off 5th and then return them to the mother store, Saks Fifth Avenue.
4. Ask and ye shall receive: question a salesperson as to when the new shipments are coming in. You can even say something specific like, "Do you expect the new Armanis this week?"

When you come home laden with great buys (don't spend more than you can afford, whatever the temptation!), you're going to dazzle the man of your dreams—whenever he shows up. In the meantime, you can wear your new treasure to next week's party, where true love may just be waiting.

Here's Another Tip:
Have You Ever Tried an Online Discount Store?

The Internet offers instant access to high-end, this-season merchandise at greatly lowered prices, takes your money right then and there, and then delivers the goods. Here's how it works. Know what you want before you even go online. (Canvass the department stores and jot down items and retail prices—e.g., Kenneth Jay Lane purse, $170; Delman shoes, $195; etc.) Then, go online and type in the name of the online discount store. My favorite is *Bluefly.com,* but you can try *Overstock.com, CoolStuffCheap.com, Ashford.com,* and any one of a hundred online discount stores. Enter the item you're looking for, and if it's in stock, you can order it right then and save yourself the hassle of on-site shopping (although I personally adore on-site shopping). Often the company picks up postage and delivery fees. If the particular item is not available, you'll see photographs of hundreds of alternatives—all at hefty discounts. At one such online store, for example, I purchased Gucci sunglasses for $139—which was 56 percent off the retail price. **Star tip:** When you locate an item online, jot down the style, name, manufacturer or designer, and basically anything that specifies it. Then put these search words into a search engine (yahoo.com or google.com for example) and compare the prices. Check out the different stores, their ratings and reviews and choose the best deal. It takes time but it will save you lots of money.

Full-Figure Fashion Finds

Okay, now remember the goal isn't to be skinny, it's to be healthy, and for some of us, healthy is a size 16 or 18. Like me, you might need a few resources with chic clothing sized for the full-figured, healthy body. First, let me address the fact that the average American woman is a size 12 or better. Many retailers have seen this demographic as their potential customer and have upped their existing product size ranges to include 16–22.

But what about making a truly positive commitment to American women by offering an outstanding and more complete line of apparel and accessories?

Women with Rubenesque curves usually don't have a destination shop in their neighborhoods that caters to the fun-loving, bold, and beautiful women we really are. We need a place to shop where we can get head-to-toe fashion for work, play, and those Sundays when we just want to take it easy. You know I'm working on it, sisters, so keep a look out for my next big move, but in the meantime, here's what I've found:

❖ I've always discovered great stuff at Lane Bryant and Ashley Stewart stores. Lane Bryant is the only place a full-sized woman can get a good strapless at a reasonable price. In fact, every single pair of underwear I've worn from age sixteen until forty-one came from Lane Bryant. (I know . . . too much information.)

❖ I've also found good choices in catalogs and online at www.newport-news.com (good bathing suits), www.barriepace.com, and at www.bluefly.com.

❖ Many of the stores mentioned as outlet centers have small sections for full-figured women. Certainly, Loehmann's, Saks Fifth Avenue's Off 5th, and other large outlets often have designer clothing especially tailored to larger sizes. Call and ask. I lived in Off 5th when I was a size 22. I may have been big but I still wanted to look good.

❖ Don't forget to check out the resources on AOL and at Amazon.com as they also have great lists.

Shopping Abroad

I wish someone had hooked me up the way I'm about to hook you up.

Outlets abound almost everywhere. Before you leave for foreign shores, you can check out any country or city on the Internet (for example, just type in London—outlet shopping) and write down the information. In fact, wherever you are, pull out the language dictionary of the region and look up "outlet shopping" or "bargain shopping" and, in the native language, ask your concierge to write down the address and point you in the right direction.

Always telephone before heading off to a foreign outlet to make sure it's still in business and still at the address you have. You might also ask what special merchandise is available. If the outlets listed below don't have a telephone number, none was available at press time. The concierge in your hotel will help you (or try the telephone book). Then, give the concierge a tip. It's worth it.

If you happen to go on a trip abroad and you want to do a little shopping Star's way, here are my special finds.

You can tip me later.

Star's Guide to the Best International Outlet Shopping

England

✳ *McArthurGlen Designer Outlets*

See Web site for locations
+44 (0) 207 535 2300
www.mcarthurglen.com
Brands: These outlets feature a variety of designers like Armani, Ben Sherman, Burberry, Calvin Klein, Paul Smith, Polo Ralph Lauren, Ted Baker, and Yves Saint Laurent.
Star tips: McArthurGlen is an excellent designer outlet chain with locations throughout Europe (several in the United Kingdom, others in France, Italy, Holland, and Austria) where you can find discounts of up to 50 percent. My two favorite ones are listed under Italy: Castel Romano and Serravalle.

London　London has a great range of shopping. Here are some of my favorite outlets:

✳ *Burberry Factory Shop*

29-53 Chatham Place
Hackney, London
+44 20 8985 3344
Mon–Fri 11–6, Sat 10–5, Sun 11–5
Brands: Burberry.
Star tips: Located on the outskirts of East London in Bethnal Green, this outlet is worth the trip. Burberry is always a great investment, as their styles are classic, classy, and timeless. Here you'll find their pieces for 50 percent off the retail price.

✳ *Designer Warehouse Sales*

45 Balfe Street
London
+44 020 7837 3322
www.designerwarehousesales.com
Check Web site for days and hours
Brands: Vary according to season, but always an outstanding collection of high-end designers. Past designer labels have included Jil Sander, Dolce & Gabbana, Nigel Preston, as well as new designers like Hussein Chalayan.
Star tips: Named The Best Designer Discount outlet in London by the *Independent,* by *Time Out London* as one of the Ten Best Reasons for living in London, and by *Elle* as a Top Twenty favorite shopping spot. There's usually a nominal entrance fee, but once inside it's worth it for one-of-a-kinds from designer shows, showroom samples, and canceled orders from the season's collections. Sales are held twelve times a year for three days at a time. Please don't miss these sales . . . it will greatly disturb me.

Italy

Florence Florence's outskirts (about forty-five minutes from the city center) are full of factory outlets where you can get up to 50 percent discount on their goods.

✳ *The Mall Outlet Center*

Via Europa 8
50060 Leccio, Reggello—Firenze
+39 055 865 77 75
+39 055 865 78 01
Mon—Sat 10–7, Sun 3–7
Brands: Sergio Rossi, Prada, D&G, Fendi, Loro Piana, Bottega Veneta, Emanuel Ungaro, Ermenegildo Zegna, Giorgio Armani, Gucci, Hogan, La Perla, Salvatore Ferragamo, Tod's, Valentino, Yves Saint Laurent, MaxMara, and Miu Miu.
Star tips: It's worth the trip outside of Florence (you'll have to either sign up for a tour bus, hire a taxi to take you out there, or take the train and then a taxi), but the selection, quality, and discounts found at these stores are unbeatable anywhere else in the world. If you're anywhere even remotely near Florence, take the time to visit these outlets. I rode right past the Leaning Tower of Pisa and got the best bargains of my shopping life. I literally lost my mind here one summer!

✳ *Space Outlet Store*

Località Levanella
52025 Montevarchi
+39 055 919 01
+39 055 978 94 81
Usually open daily, but call to check
Brands: Prada, Miu Miu, Jil Sander, Helmut Lang, Church shoes.

Star tips: Arrive early at this store, as tourist buses start arriving at about 11 a.m., and the best pieces go early. Also, if you arrive later, you'll most likely have to wait in line, as only a certain number of people are allowed into the store at one time. If you come on the weekends, holidays, and peak sale periods, prepare to be annoyed and frustrated. But it still may be worth it because you can hit Space and The Mall (above) in the same day.

＊ *Raffaelle Buccioni*

403/D Via Aretina
+39 055 690013
Brands: This small shoe factory is just outside of Florence. It produces beautifully crafted shoes that are sold at Neiman Marcus and Bergdorf Goodman. There is a small selection for sale in the outlet shop above the factory.
Star tips: Call first to be sure there are items currently for sale.

＊ *Fendi Outlet*

Via Pian dell'Isola 66/33
Rignano Sull'Arno
+39 055 834 981
Mon–Sat 9:30–6:30, Sun 2:20–6:20
Brands: Fendi, Celine, and Loewe.
Star tips: Call ahead to check opening hours as they are subject to sudden changes. It's hit or miss at this outlet, but the hits got me three baguette purses at less than $300 apiece when they were originally over $1,200 each!

＊ *Dolce & Gabbana Outlet Store*

Località S. Maria Maddalena, 49
Pian dell'Isola

Incisa in Val d'Arno
+39 055 833 1300
fax +39 055 833 1301
Mon–Sat 9–7, Sun 3–7
Brands: Dolce & Gabbana.
Star tips: Dolce & Gabbana and Fendi are on the same street despite the
different ways of describing the location. So don't miss it . . . you never
know.

Milan "The fashion capital of the world" is no lie. Finding great deals,
however, requires a little detective work here. The best discount shopping is
found outside the city. Read on.

✳ *Spaccio Etro*

Via Spartaco, 6
+39 02 57931
fax +39 02 5410 8539
Mon 3–7; Tue–Sat 10–1:45, 2:45–7; Sun 10–1
Brands: Etro.
Star tips: A great store! Paisley prints and high-quality silks, cashmeres,
and cottons are what Etro has become known for. Here you can find
fabrics, accessories, and clothes from past seasons at 50 percent off.
I wore Etro to the 2005 Daytime Emmys, and it's one of my favorite
dresses of all time.

✳ *McArthurGlen Designer Outlets*

Via della Moda 1
15069 Serravalle Scrivia
+39 0143 609000
http://serravalle.mcarthurglen.it
Daily 10–8

Brands: Armani, Burberry, Cacharel, Marina Yachting, Nike, Ralph Lauren, Samsonite, Sergio Tacchini, Stefanel, Valextra, and Versace.
Star tips: Some of the best deals here are on Valextra bags, where you can find them up to 50 percent off. I love my white Valextra luggage, and if you can get it half off . . . my goodness.

Rome

Rome is a wonderful city to explore. These are my favorite bargain stores:

✳ *Bulgari*

Via Condotti 10 (near Piazza di Spagna)
00187 Rome
+39 06 69 62 61
fax +39 06 678 34 19
www.bulgari.com
Brands: Bulgari.
Star tips: While not an outlet store, this is a must-see. As Fodor's travel guide puts it, "What Cartier is to Paris, Bulgari is to Rome." Bulgari represents the ultimate in Italian luxury. Prices range from the affordable to the insane, but it's worth browsing (and splurging).

✳ *Diffusione Tessile (outside of Rome in Pomezia)*

+39 069 105 673
www.diffusionetessile.it
Mon 3:30–7:30, Tue–Sat 10–7:30, Sun closed
Brands: MaxMara, Zegna.
Star tips: This is an excellent outlet. You can find a lot of deals for under 100 euros. This store stocks all MaxMara lines from Sport Max through Marina Rinaldi, but everything has been relabeled with the generic "Intrend." Don't be put off. Who sees the label once you have it on anyway?

✳ *Di Nicola*

Viale Mazzini 159
Mon 3:30–7:30, Tue-Sat 9–1, 3:30–7:30, Sun closed
Brands: Great designer brands like Cerruti, Loro Piana, Laura Biagiotti, and Versace.
Star tips: Usually the discounts are between 40 percent and 50 percent.

✳ *Discount System*

Via del Viminale 35
+39 064 746 545
Brands: Azzedine Alaïa, Ralph Lauren, Rifat Ozbek, and Prada.
Star tips: They have an excellent selection of shoes, belts, scarves, and sweaters. When I was a bit bigger, I spent a great deal on the accessories because the clothing in a lot of European outlets really didn't fit my body.

✳ *Il Discount delle Firme*

Via dei Serviti 27 (Largo del Tritone)
+39 064 827 790
Brands: Designers vary according to stock.
Star tips: This is a small store, but you can find discounts of up to 50 percent off the original retail price for famous designers as well as handbags, luggage, shoes, gloves, umbrellas, perfume, and lingerie.

✳ *Discount dell'Alta Moda*

Via di Gesù e Maria 16
Rome (near Piazza del Popolo)
+39 063 613 796
Brands: Stock varies.
Star tips: It's the luck of the draw, but discounts can be good and you can find the occasional amazing piece here.

✳ *Moda Doc*

Società Bezabea
Via B. Gosio 116
00191 Roma
+39 063 338 207

Brands: Genny, Iceberg, Prada, Versace, Complice, Sergio Rossi, and Anna Sui.

Star tips: The best deals are pieces from last season, which are the most heavily discounted. For my full-figured sisters, you'll also be able to find sizes up to size 18!

✳ *Vesti a Stock*

Via Germanico 170/A
Roma

Brands: Armani, Mani, Krizia, Trussardi, Moschino, Dolce & Gabbana, and MaxMara.

Star tips: This place is great for finding larger sizes—you can find up to size 16 in designer labels at 50 percent off.

Switzerland

✳ *FoxTown Factory Stores*

Via Maspoli 18
CH-6850 Mendrisio (near Milan)
+41 848 828 888
www.foxtown.ch/mendrisio/us/welcome.html
Daily 11–7

Brands: Dolce & Gabbana, Etro, Ferre, Gianni Versace, Gucci, Just Cavalli, Missoni, Miu Miu, Prada, Valentino. FoxTown outlet mall, just

over the Swiss/Italian border. With over forty stores, FoxTown is a
European rarity: an American-style outlet mall.

Star tips: Italians cross the border to buy Italian brands here and to take
advantage of the discounts. The average discount is anywhere between
30 percent and 70 percent. There are two other locations in Switzerland,
in Villenueve and Zurich.

Japan

❋ *Gotemba Premium Outlets (in the Tokyo area)*

1312, Fukasawa
Gotemba-shi, Shizuoka-ken
+81 0550 81 3122
www.premiumoutlets.co.jp/gotemba
Hours vary by season. Check the outlet's Web site.

Brands: 165 stores, including Lanvin, Laura Ashley, Anna Molinari, Loro
Piana, Armani, Marina Rinaldi, Bottega Veneta, Chloe, Paul & Joe, Paul
Smith, Diffusione Tessile, Escada, Etro, Theory, Kate Spade, Vivienne
Westwood, Yves Saint Laurent Rive Gauche, Sergio Rossi, and Gucci.

Star tips: At the foot of Mt. Fuji is an amazingly beautiful place for
shopping. Added bonus: there are amusement park rides for the kids so
they don't have to shop till they drop.

❋ *Rinku Premium Outlets (near Osaka)*

3-28, Rinku-ourai-minami
Izumisano City, Osaka
+81 0724 58 4600
www.premiumoutlets.co.jp/rinku
Daily 10–8

Brands: 150 stores, including Armani, Bally, BCBG Max Azria, Coach,

Dolce & Gabbana, Etro, Furla, Kookai, Marina Rinaldi, Marella, Miss Sixty, Salvatore Ferragamo, Theory, Jill Stuart, Lanvin, and Versace.

Star tips: This is one of the largest outlet malls in Japan. It can get very crowded with both locals and tourists, but the selection is excellent and remember Marina Rinaldi has plus sizes!

✴ *Sano Premium Outlets (in Sano)*

www.premiumoutlets.co.jp/sano
+81 0283 20 5800
Jan.-June 10–8
July-Aug. 10–9
Sept.-Dec. 10–8

Brands: Over 100 stores, including Lacoste, Lanvin, Bally, Paul Smith, Escada, Sisley, and Theory.

Star tips: Modeled after an early American village with shopping "streets" and "squares" evoking an eighteenth-century New England steeple. Fifty miles north of Tokyo, it's in an area where you can shop or ski at resorts near Nikko and Nasi-Kogen. Skip the skiing and buy something cute for après-ski.

✴ *Toki Premium Outlets (near the Nagoya area)*

www.premiumoutlets.co.jp/toki
+81 0572 53 3160
Mon-Fri, Sun 10–8; Sat 10–9

Brands: Lacoste, Bally, Versace, Bruno Magli, Coach, Furla, and Versace.

Star tips: Built in the image of a Colorado ski village surrounded by the mighty Rockies. It's great fun to shop in these out-of-the-ordinary surroundings.

❋ *Tosu Premium Outlets (in the Fukuoka area)*

www.premiumoutlets.co.jp/tosu
+81 0942 87 7370
Sat, Sun 10–8; Mon-Fri 10–9
Brands: 90 stores, including BCBG Max Azria, Miss Sixty, Escada Sport, Sisley, Theory, Coach, and Furla.
Star tips: Women will be happy with this one. Lots of great bargains.

Mexico

❋ *Premium Outlets Punta Norte*

Hacienda Sierra Vieja No. 2
Lotes No. 2 y No. 14
Col. Hacienda del Parque
Cuautitlán Izcalli
Estado de México
www.premiumoutlets.com.mx
Sun–Thur 11–8; Fri, Sat 11–9
Brands: Christian Dior, Coach, DKNY, Tommy Hilfiger, Pepe Jeans London, Zara, United Colors of Benetton, and Zegna.
Star tips: Here you can find discounts of 25 percent to 65 percent on in-season and first-quality merchandise.

❋   ❋   ❋

I know, I know . . . I'm a goddess and a lifesaver and a true girlfriend. Just pick me up a Prada bag at a discount and we'll call it even. Just kidding! But please visit me (www.starjones.com) and tell me of your finds.

Makeup

The best thing is to look natural, but it takes makeup to look natural.

CALVIN KLEIN

Who did it? Well, for one, Cleopatra did it. She did it a lot. Also Jezebel, Nefertiti, Clara Bow, Princess Pignatelli, Queen Latifah, Lena Horne, Jackie Kennedy, even Laura Bush. Definitely Nicole Kidman. Definitely Halle Berry.

Who didn't do it? Eleanor Roosevelt. Queen Anne. Cotton Mather's wife. Probably Mary Todd Lincoln. Lindsay Lohan when she was eleven. Lots of others didn't. Wouldn't. Couldn't.

Do what? Face painting, that's what. Otherwise known as makeup.

Down through the ages, makeup has had its ins and outs. The ancient Egyptians wouldn't be caught embalmed without a pot of black kohl (neither would I), and Roman beauties used barley flour to camouflage their classic Roman pimples. But makeup was sinful for Puritans and Englishwomen of the sixteenth century, who were subject to a law saying "a woman who seduced any one of Her Majesty's subjects by using face paint and false hair" was guilty of witchcraft. Clearly, I would have been burned at the stake.

Even the Bible comes down hard on makeup wearers, saying, "the assembly shall stone them . . . and burn up their houses with fire." Bit of an overreaction, even if it is the Bible, if you ask me.

Nevertheless, even in the most prudish of times, women have always found ways to color their faces with oils, lubricants, the color from natural berries and earth pigments, and by just pinching their own cheeks to raise some color.

Why? Because makeup helps you look terrific on your journey to finding love. Makeup, whether he knows it or not, is a definite turn-on for Prince Charming. You say your boyfriend likes the natural look? As in Gwyneth Paltrow, Holly Robinson Peete, Sheryl Crow, and the girl next door? Truth is, I could probably scrape three pounds of Bobbi Brown foundation off the face of any of those "natural-looking" women—maybe even four pounds from the girl next door.

If you want to be your most gorgeous, go to the nearest good cosmetic counter in a large department store on a day when they're doing free makeovers (this happens almost every day), and get your face done by someone who's good at it. You don't even have to buy anything, although the makeup artists appreciate it if you spring for at least a lipstick. Makeup is your friend. It gives you the strength you get from feeling pretty. It helps make you the best you can be, physically. Makeup is fun, child. In fact, I even remember my pastor encouraging all the women in church to wear our prettiest clothes and best makeup on Sundays. He told us that when we go out on Saturday night, we try to make ourselves look as good as we can, so why don't we do the same thing when we come into God's house? I don't personally believe you should come to church looking like a painted lady because you're not trying to seduce the minister, but if a little blush makes you smile, and a great lipstick perks up your face, something tells me that God doesn't find you a harlot.

Okay, walking into this section, understand I have great skin. It comes from my eighty-six-year-old grandmother, Pauline, and my mother, Shirley. I didn't do anything to deserve it—I just lucked out. But I have to tell you—as good as my skin looks when I wake up in the morning, all natural and warm from sleep, it looks better with makeup.

I love makeup. And so, secretly, do you. I know this because women who hate themselves for caring so much, who consider themselves beyond the falseness of blusher and foundation, will break the knees of any other woman who gets in front of her at the makeup artist's counter—the artist who said he'll show her how to make her eyes look larger. If you're getting ready for love, making yourself the best you can be, a little makeup never hurts.

Here's my routine:

A Star Makeup Regimen

First of all, I drink about ten to twelve glasses of water each day. I'm not exaggerating about this—there is *nothing* like water for the skin.

I always use a moisturizing cream in the day that's not too heavy and a more substantial cream at night before I go to sleep. It softens the skin and helps the next day's foundation blend over the surface. If I'm in an expensive mood, I use

La Mer or *La Prairie* Skin Caviar, which are two of the most expensive creams on the planet. When I'm in my cheapy-cheap mood, I use *Dove* moisturizing cream from the drugstore. Result—*shhhhh*—about the same.

Foundation comes next: I use *Era* Face Spray-on Foundation for all-over coverage and *Dermablend* to cover my full face of freckles. I also sometimes use the *MAC* and *Iman* brands for those days when I'm toning down the diva. Like most people's, my skin has different colors, so I often use two colors to enhance the natural variations on my face. I use a lighter color under my eyes, along the nose, and at the forehead. Then, with a darker color, I blend the foundation until it all melds together. I top with the number 5 face powder from *Yves Saint Laurent*.

Eye makeup comes next. I blend my own *Star Jones* colors (or I use *MAC*) on my eyelids, and I use potted black kohl along the eye line. I must say, I love to experiment with color, often combining five shades on my lids—blended well; a streak of blue, then a streak of gold is pretty tacky. After the eyelid color, I put on my fake eyelashes because my own lashes are very thin. They attach with a special glue, but I always use mascara on the top and the bottom eye line to really connect those lashes with the eye rim. I can put my lashes on in the back of a fast-moving car.

By the way, it's pretty impossible to wear false eyelashes made of mink and not have everyone notice. Jennifer Lopez somehow managed this at the 2001 Academy Awards with her see-through dress.

Then, I apply a powder blusher in soft brush puffs of a rosy or amber tone along the cheekbone. I still suck in my cheeks and then go above that "suck line" to find the right place—then blend, blend, blend. Good blending is the secret to all wonderful makeup.

Lips next. I use a lip liner that's just a shade darker than the lipstick I plan to wear—less is more when it comes to lip liner—and after applying the lipstick, I blend the liner into the color with a small brush. You don't want a Bozo the Clown lip liner—that's so 1980s. A little *MAC* lip gloss finishes off the mouth.

Brows: I use something called Brow Fix from *MAC*. It comes in a brush applicator in many colors, almost like mascara for eyebrows. It lifts and smoothes my brows (which I've already had waxed or tweezed by my makeup artist, in a "brow lift.")

At the end of the day, I remove my eyeliner and mascara with a all-one makeup remover (usually MAC). I tend to have sensitive eyes, and I get a buildup of old products if I don't cleanse my face well. I then remove the makeup with an all-in-one makeup remover and clean my face with Noxzema, La Mer, or Dove cleanser.

Get this: I never use soap. Before I go to sleep, I clean my face with *Huggies* Baby Wipes (I like the ones with aloe and vitamin E). I figure if it's good enough for a baby's butt, it's good enough for my face. My latest find is *Noxzema* Wet Cleansing Cloths, and they're also terrific (Vivica A. Fox turned me on to these). The cloths actually have Noxzema (you know, that old standby cream in the blue jar that worked for your momma and mine) in wipe form, packed and ready for travel.

Do I do this religiously? No, ma'am. I'd be lying if I told you I did it every single night of my life. Sometimes, if my makeup looks really good (like when the great makeup artist Jay Manuel from "America's Next Top Model" does it for a photo shoot or a walk on the red carpet), I want to save it for the next day, so I do without the night-before process. It hasn't killed me yet. Even though Al says on those nights I look like a cadaver painted with lashes and all, sleeping like a baby.

And that's it, from my perspective. Now, what about you?

Tips from a Master

We've all got different complexions, needs and preferences in makeup, and rather than suggest generic advice on specific problems which you can find in any good book devoted exclusively to makeup (there are tons on the shelves), I want to offer some general suggestions from one of the most astute icons in the beauty business—the late Estée Lauder herself. My friend journalist Sherry Suib Cohen interviewed Mrs. Lauder before her death, and the tips she offered are worth their weight in gold. Estée felt from the bottom of her heart that pride in one's appearance was as important as pride in one's intelligence. Here are some Lauderisms:

⁘ Lips are to kiss. Look at yours closely; they aren't only one shade of color, right? For the most kissable lips, use two shades which add more texture, depth, and lusciousness than just one. A tender mouth, for example, could have coral as an underlying shade with a soft red or pink over it. Then, a subtle gloss in a natural or even copper shade, *just on the lower lip,* makes those lips irresistibly kissable. The one shade a mouth should never be is dark brown; nothing is more aging.

✦ Color is important at the corners and edges of the mouth: don't let your lipstick fade away. As women age, their mouths seem less distinct: make yours young and defined.

✦ Buy foundation in a shade that's slightly *lighter* than your natural skin color. A darker shade will stain imperfections and make them more visible.

✦ If you have tiny wrinkles or creases on your eyelids, frosted anything will draw attention to them.

✦ Blusher should be brushed onto the places where you naturally blush (chin and forehead), not just on the suck-in spot of your cheekbones.

✦ Broken blood vessels, blemishes, prominent veins, and anything else you want to hide can be muted by dabbing some concealing cream on the area and blending it in, *before* applying your foundation. Remember—experience and time may bring more lines, but they also bestow more vitality and depth on a face. Concealer can make tired-looking undereye puffs less visible; apply the cream in dots under the puff (never on it), and blend gently with fingertips. And those puffs can magically decrease if you lie down for a few moments with some cheap, wet teabags (the cheap ones have more tannic acid, which reduces puffiness) on and under your closed eyes.

✦ Drink, drink, drink water, especially on an airplane—one glassful for every hour of flying because the skin aspirates so much moisture. Ignore the wine; alcohol is a vasodilator (it relaxes and widens blood vessels, making them visible), so one drink at 30,000 feet is like three drinks—crummy for skin.

✦ Contour (color that adds interest to your face by digging out cheekbones, even where there are none) goes *under* the cheekbone, not on top of it; feel your face and pay attention to the hollow under the cheekbone. Brush on (with a great sable brush) the rusty brownish powder in the hollow and out from the middle of the cheek hollow to the hairline in a slanting direction. You can also lightly brush some contour down the sides of a wide nose to "narrow" it or on the underside of a chin to "paint out" chin sag or double chins. Blend, blend, blend over any place you've applied contour with translucent powder for a professionally finished look.

❋ If you're a blonde, you need more makeup at night than your darker sister. "Blondes fade out at night," Estée Lauder used to say. "More glow" was her advice.

❋ Save the killer makeup (the dramatic, sometimes glittery but never gloppy stuff), almost always the evening makeup, for when you go to see the queen, have a date to meet a fabulous new guy, are on your way to the beautiful-people cocktail party, or are hosting your own stylish dinner at home. Killer makeup should be savored like a fine wine and never worn on the tennis court.

❋ How to make your makeup last:

  · Powder your lid with translucent powder before you put on your eye color.
  · Brush a bit of translucent powder on your eyelashes before applying mascara.
  · Coat your lips with foundation first, then lightly brush with translucent powder; then apply lipstick, blot, apply more powder, then more color—then, the final coat of gloss.
  · Powder blushers last longer than cream ones.

❋ *Finish* your look before you walk into the room where your lover or the whole party awaits you. Don't finish on the way in by pulling on your hair or wiping away the oil on your nose. One great way to be sure you're finished is to check your daytime makeup in the daylight; keep a mirror by the window so you can see what everyone else will see. The *six-feet test* is another good way to tell if you're finished. Stand six feet away from your mirror and slowly walk toward it. Are lips, eyes, cheeks—*anything*—jumping out, preceding your entrance? You're not finished. A great makeup is having everything on your face but looking as though you were born that way. A great makeup is *soft*.

The Budget-Beautiful Face

"Spend all you have for loveliness, / Buy it and never count the cost," wrote poet Sara Teasdale, and millions of women all over the world who can little afford it buy into this philosophy. Auntie Star's here to tell you that you can still have the most beautifully made-up face in the world, but instead of spending a fortune on it, you can have the same face on a budget.

You never need to spend a fortune on beauty products for the fabulous face that will help make an impression on Mr. Wonderful. Of course the pricey fabulous products are usually great, and you can find (and try on) your favorites at most top department stores. But I, for one, will almost always go for the very best lower-priced products, which usually can be found at any large drugstore or cosmetics outlet store.

Paula Begoun, author of *Don't Go to the Cosmetics Counter Without me* (Beginning Press, Seattle, WA, and available in bookstores and at Amazon.com) has been a guest on *The View* several times. Her philosophy (and mine) is that looking beautiful doesn't have to cost a fortune. Here are some of her (and my) suggestions for the best budget products from the drugstore and my favorite mass beauty stores like Sephora and MAC.

Drugstore Fabulous for the Face

ALL-AROUND BODY WASH: **Neutrogena**
FACIAL CLEANSERS: **Cetaphil** cleansers are constituted for dry and for normal to oily skin. **Neutrogena** puts out a great, reasonably priced product, and so does **Dove** and **Noxzema.**
MOISTURIZERS: **Dove** products (Star loves), **Avon** Botanisource

Comforting Moisture Cream, **Burt's Bees** Marshmallow Vanishing
Creme, **Kiss My Face** Vitamin C and A Ultra Rich Moisturizer,
Dr. Jeannette Graf, M.D. Skin Deep Day Facial Moisturizing Crème,
Aveeno Skin Brightening Daily Treatment SPF 15.
ACNE TREATMENT: **Clean & Clear** Persa-gel, **Clean & Clear** Sheets,
Neutrogena Pore Treatment.
TEETH WHITENERS: **Colgate** Whitening Gel, **Crest** Dental Strips,
Arm & Hammer Mint Toothpaste, **Colgate** Fluoride Toothpaste.
FOUNDATIONS: *Oily skin:* **Almay** Amazing Lasting Sheer Makeup
SPF 12, **Clinique** Superfit Makeup, **Black Opal** True Color Liquid
Foundation Oil-Free, **Maybelline** EverFresh Makeup SPF 14.
Normal to oily/combination skin: **Avon** beComing Redefine Airbrush
Foundation SPF10, **CoverGirl** Fresh Look Oil-Free Makeup SPF 15,
Neutrogena Visibly Firm Moisture Makeup SPF 20, **L'Oréal** True Match
Super-Blendable Makeup.
Normal to dry skin: **The Body Shop** Oil-Free Face Base, **Almay** Skin
Smoothing Foundation with Kinetin SPF 15, **Revlon** Age Defying
Makeup with Botafirm SPF 20, **MAC** Studio Finish Matte Foundation
SPF 8.
Extra dry skin: **Avon** Face Lifting Moisture Firm Foundation Cream
Soufflé, **Origins** Dew Gooder Moisturizing Face Makeup.
EYE CIRCLE DEPUFFER: **Olay** Regenerist Eye Lifting Serum.
EYELINERS: **Almay** Amazing I-Liner Liquid Eyeliner, **Clinique** Eye
Defining Liquid Liner, **Bonne Bell** Eye DeFiner pencil, **Maybelline**
Expert Eyes Defining Liner, **Rimmel** Exaggerate Full Color Eye Definer
pencil, **MAC** Fluidline.
EYE SHADOWS: **Avon** True Color powder eyeshadows, **Laura Mercier**
powder eye shadows, **Revlon** Illuminance Creme Shadow, **Stila** Shadow
Pots, **MAC** powder eye shadow.
ANTIWRINKLE CREAM: **Almay** Kinetin Rejuvenating Eye Treatment.
CONCEALER: **Max Factor** Erace, **CornSilk** Liquid Powder Con-
cealer.
BLUSHER: **Almay** Nearly Naked Touch-Pad Blush, **Face Stockholm**
powder blush, **MAC** powder blush.

BRONZER: **MAC** Bronzing Powder, **Nars** Blush-Bronzer Duo. (Sephora has these.)

MASCARA: **L'Oréal** Lash Intensifique; **Maybelline** Lash Expansion, and Wonder Curl Waterproof; **Sonia Kashuk** Lashify; **Revlon** ColorStay Lashcolor; **Rimmel** Extra Super Lash; **CoverGirl** Professional Waterproof, **Shu Uemura** mascara.

FALSE EYELASHES: **Shu Uemura.**

LIPSTICK: **Aloette** Lip Color, **Clinique** Long Last Soft Shine, **Wet 'n' Wild** MegaPlump.

LIP GLOSS: **Wet 'n' Wild** MegaSlicks Lip Gloss, **Aveda** Lip Shine, **MAC** lip gloss.

LIP LINER PENCILS: **Aloette** Waterproof Mechanical LipDefiner Pencil, **Merle Norman** Definitive Lip Liner, **N.Y.C.** Lipliner Pencil.

MAKEUP BRUSHES: **Stila, MAC, Sonia Kashuk.**

CREAM HAIR-REMOVAL: **Nair** and **Surgi-Cream** depilatories.

EYEBROW TWEEZERS: **Tweezerman** products.

MAKEUP REMOVER: **Dove** Daily Hydrating Cleansing Cloths, **Estée Lauder** Gentle Eye Makeup Remover, **Origins** products; **Lancôme** Bi-Facil, **Noxzema** products.

Fabulous but More Pricey

BEST PIMPLE HEALER	*Kiehl's* Blue Herbal Spot Treatment
BEST MOISTURIZERS	*Clinique* Dramatically Different Moisturizing Gel
	Chanel Précision Hydramax + Moisture Boost Cream
BEST FACIAL CLEANSER	*Purpose* Gentle Cleansing Wash
BEST LIQUID FOUNDATION	*La Mer* The Foundation
	Giorgio Armani Luminouse Silk Foundation
BEST MASCARA	*T. LeClerc* Waterproof Mascara
	Lancôme Flextencils

BEST BODY LOTION   *Clarins* Energizing Hydra-Wear Express Body Lotion

BEST COMPACT MAKEUP   *Clinique* Superbalanced Compact Makeup SPF 20

BEST LIP GLOSS   *DiorKiss* Lip Gloss

Ten Beauty Products Star Can't Live Without

Every beauty expert has a list of favorites. Here's mine:

1. **Maybelline** Great-Lash Mascara and false eyelashes!
2. **Neutrogena** Deep Clean Facial Cleanser or Noxzema Daily Cream Cleanser
3. **MAC** "Oh Baby" Tinted Lipglass
4. **Yves Saint Laurent** Semi Loose Powder
5. **Huggies Unscented** Baby wipes
6. **"Jiffy Tan"** body lotion by benefit
7. **La Prairie** Skin Caviar Luxe Cream or La Mer Crème da la Mer Moisturizer
8. **Era** Face Spray-On Foundation
9. **Scott Barnes** Body Bling
10. **Iman** Luxury Pressed Powder

Hair

Blown hair is sweet.

T. S. ELIOT

Her hair shall be of what color it please God.

WILLIAM SHAKESPEARE (WRONG, WILLIAM. YOU CAME BEFORE CLAIROL)

When I was legal correspondent for NBC television, I was different from almost every other correspondent. First of all, I was young and had actually been a practicing attorney, when most of the other legal talking heads were seasoned college professors or people who had given up the practice of law a long while back. I was also a black woman, the only one, I think, in the club. And then, there was my hair.

I approached hair differently from my other female legal sisters. I treated it as an accessory, which I still do. I changed my hair as I did my earrings, shoes, and handbags. It depended on my mood and what made me feel pretty that day. I wore wigs or hairpieces almost every day—I still do. One day, I'd sport a long ponytail. Another day, I'd wear my hair sort of curly-curly. One day it was straight; one day tied back; the next day swooped to the side. Evolving, different hairstyles made me feel pretty.

One morning, an intense, sober network honcho took me aside with a very grave suggestion. "If you had a consistent hairdo, I think you'd be taken more seriously," he intoned.

I looked at him. "Consistent hairdo?" I repeated. "Ain't gonna happen."

And then, I told him that I knew more about what I was talking about than anybody listening. He knew it was true. "I think the audience can figure out what I'm saying and how seriously they should take this by what I say, not by how I wear my hair." And then, I turned around and left him and his consistency standing alone.

I refused to fit into the cookie-cutter, plain old Saltine cracker mold of what a journalist should look like. Conforming was out of the question. And that sort of became my trademark.

Now, this section is about hair, but please take this little story beyond television, beyond any profession, beyond hair. You are allowed, should you be tempted, to refuse conformity. You can work in a dental office or in Waldbaum's or be a brain surgeon and still look different from your coworkers. That's style. That's independence.

I believe that having the courage of your convictions is the truest way to prepare yourself to be the best you can be—so you'll be ready to meet your mate.

Back to hair.

Weaves, Wigs, and Wonderful Hairpieces

When I first started talking about weaves and wigs and hairpieces, it was a big deal. Now every movie star in the world adds hair extensions and little weave pieces. For that community it's newish to talk about it, but in my community, it's been a topic of conversation for a long time. I really enjoy seeing women of every color doing everything from natural braids and close-cropped hair, to wearing long extensions to their butts, like Shakira. My husband loves when my hair's long and straight—he thinks that's sexy. He also likes it when I curl it. Most of all, he likes when I shake it all up and change my look. "You've been wearing your hair like that a lot," he'll say. It's my cue that I'm getting in a rut and it would be nice to give him something a little different.

If you've learned anything at all in getting ready for the man in your life by making yourself the best you can be physically, it's this: do what feels good to you. I despise people telling me that I shouldn't wear a straight hair weave because I'm black and "you're embracing a European style of what's beautiful." Wrong. I'm embracing the Star style. If you really wanted to get technical, you'd know that all hairstyles originated back on the continent of Africa—long, short, bald, curly, and straight. Never feel ashamed to express your individuality because someone wants to put you in a box; let him stay in the box, all by himself.

Hair weaves and extensions aside, it all starts with the cut. A great haircut is the secret of really wonderful hair.

Here are some elemental tips on haircuts that are right for you from Vincent Roppatte, hairstylist to the stars and director of the Elizabeth Arden Red Door Salons at Saks Fifth Avenue stores nationwide.

How do you know if you have a great haircut?

Vincent says, "Shake your head when you're out dancing: does the hair fall back into a flattering, swingy, terrific shape? Is it bouncy, does it swirl like a river? You have a great haircut. Look in the mirror after your swim in the pool. The hair's wet, sure, but after a quick tousle with your fingers, is it still cute? You have a great haircut. Do people stop you in the street and ask, 'Who cuts your hair?' You have a great haircut."

The Fabulous Hairstylist

Here's the key to it all:

You need to find the fabulous hairstylist who will give you that perfect cut, that hair advice tailored just to your texture, the one who will make your life easy—let alone pretty.

How do you find a great hairstylist? Ask someone on the street whose look you think is stunning the following question: Who does your hair? Even if you have to stop someone at a party or ask the woman next to you on the bus, don't feel embarrassed—people love to be asked this question.

Before you let a new stylist do anything extreme, see him or her for a few appointments before you opt for the cut. Do you like what he does to your hair when he's just setting or blow-drying it? Good start. Now, on haircut day, bring him a picture of the way you want your hair to look: any great hairdresser will appreciate that. A mediocre hairdresser will feel threatened by a photograph because he probably knows he can't achieve it. A good hairstylist will also tell you why a cut would or would not look good on you.

How much should this cost? For a great cut that lasts weeks, maybe even two or three months, be prepared to mortgage your firstborn. Eat less, go to fewer sales, do anything to be thrifty, and save up for that haircut: it's money well spent. Don't let your best friend, Vanda, cut your hair, unless her name is really Mr. Vincent.

Cool Cuts for Your Face Shape

A great cut can make your month. It makes your hair easier to blow-dry and style. It takes a great hairstylist to know what's best for your face and figure—speaking of which, when you're getting a haircut, don't ignore your body shape. If you're very large, a close-cropped haircut can make you look plain silly. But mostly, at haircut time, it's the shape of the face you must consider.

No one has a perfectly round, oval, or heart-shaped face, but do you come close to any of these categories? Find out by pulling your hair back with a band. Now, standing close to a very well lit mirror, with a wet bar of soap trace the outline of your face onto the mirror. Now you know your face shape!

Remember that none of these suggestions is set in stone. You may try some color extensions that look incredibly good and break all the rules below. And if you get a haircut that is all wrong, don't freak: hair grows back.

Square Face

Who has a square-shaped face? Journalist, author, and wife of Governor Arnold Schwarzenegger, Maria Shriver has a classically square-shaped face. You have one also if your face seems wider at the jawline and forehead than the sides—almost as wide as it is long.

Try: A long cut, but gently layered. If your jaw is particularly square, ask your hairstylist for a cut that will be fuller at the top than at the bottom to deemphasize that square jaw. If your face is widest at the forehead, ask for a cut that can be fashioned fuller at the chin to deemphasize the square forehead. Medium-length bangs cut slightly shorter in the center work wonderfully. A sharp, geometric cut is *not* for you.

Heart-shaped Face

Who has a heart-shaped face? The actress Reese Witherspoon, for one. Also, Eva Longoria and Beyoncé. Lindsay Lohan comes close to a heart-shaped face. You have one also if your face has high cheekbones, a wide-ish forehead, and a pointy chin.

Try: A midlength (just past your ears) tousled shag. Or ask your hairdresser about a layered bob with extra volume near the chin: that softens your narrow, heart-shaped face. Long, tapered bangs, perhaps swept to one side, also work well. A very short haircut and a center part are *not* for you.

Oval Face

Who has an oval-shaped face? Star Jones Reynolds does. Also Alicia Keys. You have one also if your face looks more oval (egg shaped) than square, round, or long. Lucky girl. Ovals can wear any cut or style.

Try: Everything! Consider Iman's wild and wonderful shock of hair, consider the original straight, layered Jennifer Aniston look, consider a mass of long Shirley Temple curls. One of the best looks for oval? A straight, angled-at-the-jaw cut.

Narrow and Long and Angular Face

Who has such a face? Jamie Lee Curtis does. Also Brandy. You have one also if you have a high forehead and a longish chin. Long faces often have great cheekbones.

Try: A layered cut that doesn't make your hair high or full at the very top of your head: you need fullness around your face. If your hair is cut above chin length, it will make your face look even more narrow. You might try a side part (it widens the forehead and softens the length). Try wisps around the face, as well. Do *not* get a long, all-one-length cut.

Round Face

Who has a round-shaped face? Hillary Clinton's face is roundish, and so is Mandy Moore's and Isabella Rossellini's. If yours is also, you probably have chipmunk-y cheeks and they dominate your cheekbones. Your chin is wide and full.

Try: Longer hair—say, shoulder length. Make sure your hairdresser layers it with more height on top to "ovalize" the roundness. A short fringy cut brushed toward the face also works for you because it seems to narrow the face. Do *not* opt for a cut that makes your hair very full and frizzy or curly. Color can seem to change face shapes: An aureole of light hair around a long, thin face widens it. The same light-colored aureole around a round face makes it seem moon shaped. Not a great look. You can have highlights color-painted throughout your hair by your hairdresser to distract from its roundness. Color painting is simply brushing bleach in tiny areas where a frosty light-up would look great.

Some Personal Hair Tips

Have you noticed that . . .

- ✳ brushing the proverbial hundred strokes every night breaks and damages your hair? You're right—it does.
- ✳ the sudsiest shampoos are the hardest to rinse out? Also, they don't do much for cleanliness because the soap residue attracts dirt.
- ✳ the steam room's a great place to condition hair with a protein conditioner after shampooing? Steam opens hair shafts, and the conditioner penetrates more deeply.
- ✳ if you want to straighten your hair, you must use fat, round brushes? Gently pull each section of hair taut away from the roots as you dry around the fat brush; release when hair has cooled down from dryer.
- ✳ when hair is totally dry, a few strokes with a fat paddle brush further straightens it. Use the dryer set to medium heat, and paddle brush over the hair's surface from roots to tips for a straight, smooth finish.
- ✳ if you want to curl your hair, you should brush mousse or gel through wet hair? Divide the hair into small sections and hold with clips. One by one, wrap each section around the bristles of a *narrow* round brush, and blow dry. Allow each section to cool before you unroll the brush to go to the next section. For a pageboy, roll the hair under. For a flippy look, roll the hair up and over the brush.

* too often, you have errant hair, cowlicks, bangs that won't settle down? Put cellophane tape across the section of wet hair that's giving you grief until it's dry. Problem gone.

* television lights do funny things to hair? If you plan to be on TV for any reason, stay away from red highlights or red hair additions— they'll look hoochie. Try rich auburn instead.

* you always have a bad hair day when it's most important to look great? If you're planning to meet your future mother-in-law or have a first date with the guy who may be *it* and you wake up with a head full of knots, tangles, and hair going every which way, try these:

  · Stunning, oversize shades pushed back on your head contain frizzies in an emergency.

  · Tie your hair into a ponytail or sweep it up on a humid afternoon.

  · Marvelous barrettes, jeweled bobby pins, headbands, or tortoiseshell grip combs do wonders.

  · An emergency wig: try one with an attached headband. You can just roll out of bed and go.

  · If all else fails, a stunning scarf or cap can look très chic.

Show Biz Secret

A vitamin E capsule, broken open, is the world's best conditioner—even if your hair is not frizzy. Dab the contents of one 400 unit vitamin E capsule (you can mix it with one ounce of olive or soybean oil) on the ends of your hair and on any areas where your hair is damaged. Comb through and apply a warm, wet towel for twenty minutes (or sit under a heat cap, which you can buy in any beauty supply store). Then, shampoo (apply the shampoo and work into a lather before you add the water—oil and water don't mix, remember) and rinse very thoroughly.

Dish on Frizz

Everyone has frizzy hair days no matter the texture or ethnic origin of her hair. Vincent Roppatte suggests some quick fixes:

* Apply several drops of an antifrizz shine serum (like *John Frieda Frizz-Ease*) to a fat, fluffy makeup brush, and brush over your wet hair. Then, blow-dry it and slick it back with a firm-bristled, flat brush. Hold it, Grace Kelly style, with a marvelous barrette or ribbon.
* If you softly blow-dry just the hairline before you slick hair severely back, it softens the look immeasurably. Try *Wella* Lifetex Personal Trainer, another fierce frizz controller. You can combine styles especially if your hair is longer: sleek back your hair, braid it halfway down, and then leave the rest in its naturally frizzy state—an adorable look.
* A moisturizing, protein-rich shampoo (try *Paul Mitchell* Instant Moisture Daily Shampoo or any product containing shea butter) at least twice weekly.
* Get a great cut: a summertime cut by a fine stylist removes bulk, so there's less hair to frizz up.

Drugstore Fabulous for the Hair

My expert, Paula Begoun, author of *Don't Go Shopping for Hair-Care Products Without Me* (Beginning Press, Seattle, WA, and available in bookstores and Amazon.com) offers a treasure trove of hair products that won't empty your wallet.

BEST SHAMPOOS (will not cause buildup and cost $8 or less): **Breck** Beautiful Hair; **Jheri Redding** Shine Shampoo with Vitamin C for Dull, Dry Hair; **Queen Helene** Natural Garlic Shampoo, Unscented;

TRESemmé European Deep Cleansing Shampoo; **White Rain** Extra Body Shampoo; **Garnier Fructis** Fortifying Anti-Dandruff Shampoo. BEST CONDITIONERS for normal to dry hair ($8 or under): **Avon** Advance Techniques Color-Protection Conditioner; **Infusium 23** Colored/Permed Revitalizing Conditioner; **Salon Grafix** Daily Balancing Conditioner; **Prell** Spa Formula Conditioner.

BEST CONDITIONERS for dry to very dry hair ($8 or under): **L'Oréal** Nature's Therapy Mega Repair Recovery Complex; **Pantene** Full and Thick Conditioner; **Jheri Redding** Extra Humidicon Moisturizing Conditioner.

BEST STYLING PRODUCTS ($12 or less): **Bath & Body Works** Bio Curl on Cue Shine Serum; **John Frieda** Frizz Out Hair Serum; **Rusk** Thickening Spray; **Wella** Long Hair Styler; **Paul Mitchell** Light Hold Spray Gel; **Suave** Hairspray; **Aussie** Flexible Hold Styling Mist; **African Pride** Spray On Braid Shampoo; **Isoplus** No-Lye Conditioning Crème Relaxer; **Dark and Lovely** Conditioning No-Lye Relaxer System.

BEST HAIR TOOLS: **Conair** straightener; **Revlon** straightener.

BEST BRUSHES: Sonia Kashuk brushes; Denman brushes.

BEST BLOW-DRYER (use only straight-nozzle blow-dryers): **Vidal Sassoon** Professional 1875 Watt Dryer with Metal Finish; **BaByliss** professional hair dryer.

That's Paula's list. She's the expert, but come on, girls, you *know* I also know hair. Here are my . . .

Ten Hair Must-Haves

1. Electric hot rollers
2. Elgin Charles Leave-In Conditioner
3. Covered elastic (not rubber) bands
4. Ceramic flat iron
5. "Big and Sexy" hair spray

6. Aveda Anti-Humectant Moisturizer
7. Fake ponytail
8. Curling iron
9. Professional blow-dryer with diffuser
10. Emergency wig!
    (From the Star Jones Collection, www.especiallyyours.com)

So, What Do You Think?

Are you getting there—the best you can be physically? I have a feeling you're close. Now it's time to consider your emotional state.

Part Two

Be All You Can Be, Emotionally

It wasn't enough to prepare myself physically for love. I also had to deal with the interior—with the emotional Star. It will come as no surprise to you that, in some ways, this would be an even greater challenge.

But before I even start telling you about my odyssey in this area, I'd like you to assess your own readiness for love in different emotional areas. Take these self-assessment exercises, find your strong and weak points, and then we'll talk, child.

QUIZ

ARE YOUR EMOTIONS IN CHECK?

First, assess your relationships, past and present
Choose the best answer (even if the answer isn't exactly on target)

1. What kind of men do you attract?

A. Nasty, verbally abusive guys
B. Weak personalities
C. Caring, careful lovers or friends
D. Not the sharpest knives in the drawer
E. Men whom you suspect are in the relationship only for the sex

2. How long do your relationships with men generally last?

A. Two to four months
B. Six months to a year
C. Closer to two years
D. What relationships?

3. You generally trust your boyfriends:

A. About as much as you trust Bin Laden—but there's always room for change
B. Totally
C. Most of the time

4. When it comes to a relationship with your family and friends, the guys you date keep you:

A. Explaining away their moods
B. Tense
C. Proud and happy
D. Nauseous

5. Whenever you've questioned your commitment to a guy in your life, you've often thought:

A. You'd break up with him if you weren't so afraid of being alone
B. There are many men out there who'd appreciate you more and understand you better
C. That no matter what he does, you want to wake up with him on your pillow
D. About cheating

How much do you know about your present boyfriend, or even the man who once was very important to you?

His Past

6. In high school he dated:

A. I haven't the foggiest
B. Ms. Cheerleader
C. Ms. Class Intellectual
D. The sexiest girl
E. None of the above

7. As a child, if he ever ran away from home, it would be to:

A. I haven't the foggiest
B. His religious leader
C. A relative's house
D. A friend
E. None of the above

8. His relationship with his parents is/was:

A. I haven't the foggiest
B. Devoted and respectful
C. Destructive
D. Nonexistent
E. Cordial

His Present

9. Tops on his list of Worst Things That Can Happen: he'll lose

A. His money
B. His best friend
C. His self-control
D. His erection
E. You

continued

10. In his heart of hearts he wants others to regard him with:

A. Respect

B. Love

C. Admiration for his accomplishments

D. Admiration for his power

E. Fear

11. Almost every day he feels:

A. I haven't the foggiest

B. Misunderstood

C. Unappreciated

D. Successful

E. Angry at you for something

In general (choose one)

12. If someone brought home a gift/made dinner/cleaned up/said "I love you," it would almost definitely be:

A. You

B. Him

C. Your mom

D. Because the other is dying or something

13. In a conflict, generally:

A. You avoid conflict totally: it stresses you out so you withdraw and hide your feelings.

B. You raise your voice or get violent: can't help it.

C. Your partner raises his voice or gets violent: he can't help it.

D. You both have conflict-solving skills (maybe you took a course?), and you avoid mayhem.

14. How often do you spontaneously touch, hug, stroke, or kiss your partner?

A. Often

B. Rarely

C. I save it all for bed

D. Occasionally

E. Just about never

15. Regarding criticism:

A. I simply can't deal with it. I'm overly sensitive, I know.

B. When one of us criticizes the other, we usually explode and the insults fly.

C. I've been known to admit I'm wrong.

D. I hate it—but I try to hear if there's any truth in it.

Now assess your emotional and mental health

16. Are the psychological aspects of your health represented by some of the following statements? I have some of the following signs of stress at least two or three times a week: (Check those that apply.)

____ Get seriously nuts when driving in traffic behind a slow or incompetent person

____ Feel like I want to cry

____ Have a lack of interest in sex

____ Feel like I have serious enemies who want to hurt me

____ Feel very irritable

____ Can't stop thinking about my problems

____ Have trouble with my usual work routine because I'm stressed

____ Usually get pretty hostile when I'm challenged or when I lose at something

17. What do you worry about, sometimes obsessively? (Check each one that applies.)

____ Asserting myself

____ Making friends

____ Not finding a husband

____ Being rejected

____ Being criticized

____ Death, mine or a dear one

____ Feeling stupid at work

____ Losing an argument

____ My weight

____ A feeling of emptiness that's not assuaged by food

____ Never being able to forgive someone who did a crappy thing

____ Throwing a party and no one comes

____ Being at a party and almost no one speaks to me

continued

18. Circle one or several: In order to meet interesting men (as well as women), I might:

A. Advertise in a magazine that seems to concentrate on my interests
B. Hang out in a nice bar or social club
C. Volunteer at a charitable organization
D. Join an organization that deals with people in my type of business
E. Go to church, synagogue, or mosque—whatever calls me

19. Choose the creature you think you most resemble:

A. A feral cat
B. A beloved puppy
C. A shark
D. A porcupine
E. A chameleon
F. Roadkill
G. A peacock
H. A strong, fast horse

Choose your most probable response.

20. You want to be more grown-up when it comes to money matters. You'll probably:

A. Take a course in financial preparedness
B. Throw out all your credit cards and only use cash
C. Buy your home, although it's a huge financial stretch
D. Rent instead of buy your home, although you can probably take out a loan to purchase it

21. Regarding sex and dating: I think that

A. Opposites attract. The way you enlarge your thinking is with guys who are very different from you.
B. Asking people to sign a pledge of abstinence until they get married is pretty stupid and impractical; this is the twenty-first century.
C. I'd like to meet an interesting guy's mother as soon as possible in our relationship.
D. Women ought to be smart and not tell too much about themselves early in relationships. It's no one's business what you privately think.

22. Your good friend has called, raving mad at something you did (you really did do it, but she deserved it). You:

A. Hang up. You take abuse from no one.

B. Break all ties with her: she's not worth your time.

C. Offer to talk about it when you both cool off.

D. Justify yourself and explain in detail what she did to prompt your behavior.

23. Your overall picture of life is represented by which Chinese proverbs? (Check as many or none that apply to your way of thinking.)

A. Better to bend in the wind than to break.

B. Unless there is opposing wind, a kite cannot rise.

C. Hate rises like smoke around one who surpasses one's peers.

D. Wherever one finds comfort can be called home.

E. A person must despise herself before others will.

F. Love for a person must extend to the crows on his roof.

G. Whenever the water rises, the boat will rise also.

H. Life is a treadmill and I'm the hamster.

24. To eliminate emotional stress, you'd probably:

A. Take a nap.

B. Take a pill.

C. Have a coke, coffee, or candy bar to pep you up.

D. Use your mind and willpower to convince yourself you're not really stressed out.

E. Meditate.

F. Phone a friend or listen to music.

25. It's been a very bad day. The pimple burst, the dog vomited on the carpet, and the Hammering Maniac struck in your building. You will most likely:

A. Hide under the covers.

B. Have a stiff drink, then another, then another, then a chocolate sundae.

C. Make a list of all the good things in your life and why tomorrow will be a better day.

continued

SCORING

1. A=0, B=2, C=10, D=4, E=2

2. A=0, B=10, C=2, D=0

3. A=0, B=10, C=6

4. A=2, B=2, C=10, D=0

5. A=2, B=4, C=10, D=2

6. A=0; take 10 if you answered B, C, or D and are sure of it—if you're not sure, take 0. E=10 if you're sure—otherwise, take 0.

7. A=0; take 10 if you answered B, C, or D and are sure of it—if you're not sure take 0. E=10 if you're sure—otherwise, take 0.

8. A=0, B=10, C and D=0, E=5

9. A or D=0, B and C=5, E=10

10. A or B=10, C=8, D=2, E=0

11. A, B, C, E=0, D=10

12. A=6, B=10, C=0, D=0

13. A, B, C=0, D=10

14. A=10, B=2, C=0, D=4, E=0

15. A=0, B=0, C=8, D=10

16. If you checked 6–8 answers, take 0. If you checked 3–5, take 4; if you checked 2, take 7; if you checked only 1, take 8; if you checked none, take 10.

17. If you checked 8–13 answers, take 0. If you checked 5–7, take 2. If you checked 3–4, take 3. If you checked 1–2, take 5. If you checked none, take 10.

18. A and B=0, take 5 for each of C, D, or E you checked.

19. A=2 (a wild thing does not a beloved partner make), B=5 (cute you might be, but ready for an equal, loving relationship—don't think so), C=0 (do I have to spell it out?), D=0 (don't come close!), E =0 (if you disguise yourself so brilliantly, how will the man of your dreams get to know you?), F=0 (that bad, huh?), G=4 (self-esteem you may have, but is that all?—and is it enough for a relationship?), F=10 (you look mahvelous; you're powerful and loving!)

20. A and C=10, B and D=0.

21. A=0, B=0, C=10, D=0

22. A=0 (you've probably lost a pal, forever), B=0, C=10 (an emotionally cool and intelligent response), D=3

23. Take 10 for each of the following you checked:

A (An emotionally strong woman knows that the flexible bamboo will survive a storm with less damage than the mighty oak: be reasonable and bend with your loved one instead of standing obdurately straight), B (Adversity and sometimes, even enemies give us opportunity to rise higher), C (When we lose weight, get famous, or find good fortune, envy and fear often come from colleagues or friends who we thought wished us well), D (Peace in the home is the greatest comfort), E (Self-esteem is critical to success), F (no one's perfect), and G (Hang out with good, kind, intelligent people, and when they rise in the world—they'll float your boat right along).

If you checked H, take 0. Okay, this isn't a Chinese proverb, I made it up, but if it echoes your picture of life, you're not emotionally ready for true love, mama.

24. A=2, B=2, C=0, E=10. If you answered D, *subtract* 10 from your total score. You're annoying and in a state of denial. F=10—good girl!

25. A=10. Sometimes, it just makes sense to hide in a warm place and pray that everything bad goes away. B=1. This doesn't make much sense at all because you'll get nauseous. If you chose C, you get 0 because now I'm nauseous: you're too much of a Pollyanna to ring true, and emotional denial never indicates emotional readiness.

ANALYSIS: Add up your numerical responses

If you scored between 290 and 315:
You have a high emotional IQ. You're your own best friend, you have a healthy mental outlook, and realistic and positive expectations of a future with a wonderful love. You take the time to find out about people—especially the guy who could be the love of your life. You know how to tune into the essence of people close to you. Also very important is that you understand how to deal with conflict—with your best girlfriends and colleagues, as well as with a man. And most valuable, you're your own woman, emotionally and financially in charge of your life. You have the warmth, wisdom, and ability to accept a great guy's support systems, but you never allow yourself to be swallowed whole by the choices another person makes—even if you are crazy about

continued

him. You have given thought to leading the good life, and knowingly or not, have started to prepare yourself emotionally to meet your counterpart. Read further into this chapter to strengthen your resolve even further and put yourself in the best position for him to find you. Congratulations on a great score.

If you scored between 260 and 289
You are *reasonably* prepared to meet the person with whom you'll have a seriously important relationship. I know you want an intimate connection with a partner who will be always in your corner, and that will most easily happen when *you* are most ready for him—and you're not quite there yet. If you had to pick one quality that the most successful marriages share, it's that both partners are self-starters—neither one is totally and childishly dependent on the other. Each is an organized and self-appreciating person—not to mention an acutely sensitive listener. Such partners hear each other—even when the other is not speaking because they're on the same wavelength. Does this make sense to you? Good. This chapter will tell you how to think about present and your future, deal with friends (false and true), and put your financial house in order, among other things. Please read the following pages to tap more deeply into the emotional strengths hidden just below your surface.

If you scored between 230 and 259
You need some work, baby. I promise it won't be arduous and it certainly won't be boring. I'm a little worried about your emotional and mental preparedness because your score doesn't indicate a well-developed maturity in these matters. You have enormous potential so, please—read on pal, and see if you can spot some of your weaknesses.

If you scored under 230, Yikes.
This isn't the best score on the planet. You're missing a lot of emotional nuances that aren't spelled out in ten-foot-tall letters. You *need* your Auntie Star: I promise you'll emerge far more emotionally and practically sound after you finish this book. Confession: I probably would have scored this low before I started my odyssey toward physical, emotional, and spiritual preparedness, but look at me now, baby—I'm soaring! And you will too.

*   *   *

Chapter 4

I'm Worth Everything

Protect yourself so that nobody overrides you, overrules you, or steps on you.
You just say, "Just a minute, I'm worth everything, dear."

MAYA ANGELOU

Maya is talking self-esteem here. This is the hub around which all emotional development flows. Self-esteem is liking yourself and giving yourself credit for who you are and the good things you do. You have to believe you're worthy. And that is a really hard thing to do even for women who look like they have everything.

My girlfriend and cohost on *The View* is Elisabeth Hasselbeck, and she has a tendency not to be able to take a compliment. You say to this smart, funny, beautiful woman, "Oh, you look so pretty," and the first thing out of Elisabeth's mouth is, "But my hair looks really crappy." And she means it. So, the first step toward self-esteem is to believe you look good. Believe you smell good. Believe you're smart. If all objective evidence points to the fact that you're worthy of the prince, believe you are worthy of the prince.

Here's how you collect some of that objective evidence: make a list of what's good about you—don't just read these lines, do it, right now. You can start with the silly and go to the serious. If you have beautiful hair, write

My hair is gorgeous

If you have lovely eyes, write

My eyes send people over the moon

When someone is in need, are you the first to volunteer help? Do children like you? Are you an adventurer, willing to take risks and try new things? Do you share easily? Are you kind? Did you send a donation to the animal rescue fund during the New Orleans tragedy? Are you somehow sure inside that you have the qualities that could enable a great relationship with Prince Charming—even if you've never before had such a relationship? Are you funny? Do you keep going even when you feel blue? If you can answer any of these (and your own) questions in the positive, put it on your list. Do you end up with at least seven things that are good about you? Honey, you're a terrific person—and so ready to find love!

It's been my experience that some women have been taught to feel bad about themselves, even by well-meaning mothers, fathers, sisters, friends. I was lucky—I've never been taught anything but "you're fabulous and can achieve anything you want." If you haven't been so fortunate, you've got to find your self-esteem from within yourself—because the wrong views of others won't do it for you. A long time ago I heard a song from the artist Julia Fordham where she says she's her own "tower block." Interpreting a tower block as an inner strength that stands and reaches high, and blocks out all negative light and feelings of worthlessness, Fordham says she's her own shining light, her own solid foundation, and her own energy—she pumps herself up when outside influences conspire to attack her self-esteem. I also remember reading stories about Olympic athletes who were homeless and slept in cars and were never taught to feel good about themselves; these winners became their own tower blocks as they figured out that if no one else cheered for them, they'd have to be their own cheerleaders. If the people around you put doubt into your mind, shake it off, shake it off: don't listen to those who tell you to change the way you do your hair or wear your clothes—if you like it.

Look—if you assess yourself and truly find you're lacking something, of course, try to fix it. For example, if you have a dental problem and your teeth are black or crooked, you really might have a tough time until you get those teeth fixed. But if you're getting negative comments from others about shortcomings, figure out if the comments are true or if they derive from someone who's mean-spirited, narcissistic, or who has an agenda that's not in your best interest. It's sadly true that even people who love you can be wrong. Suppose you were gangly when you were eleven and your mom constantly was at you to eat more or dress differently to hide the gangliness. Those comments dug away at your self-esteem and they still do: you can weigh two hundred pounds and still feel gangly inside. But maybe your mom had her own issues. Maybe she was just wrong when she said you looked awful the way you were. Maybe you were a gangly, adorable teenager—but mom's own problems couldn't let her see that. Shake her off, even today, shake her off, accept that she was wrong. Treat critical people as if you were a sponge. Soak up the good and wring out the bad. Bottom line: if others have advice for you, but it's not going to be useful, shake it off.

In the end, building self-esteem is really a matter of nurturing yourself—that's the best way to grow as good as you can be emotionally during your journey to make your life as good as it gets, and ultimately find true love. Approach your life as though you were blessed to be living it. I mean that.

Suppose you're a toll taker, and when people ask you, "What do you do?" you hate to answer because you secretly think you have the most boring job in the world. But what if you nurture yourself by changing the way you look at your life? What if you *will* yourself to believe you have a fascinating job—the stuff of novels? What if you look at every person who drives through that toll stop as someone who's interesting, someone who has a story. Think of those drivers as a *Desperate Housewives* plot. On the surface of Wisteria Lane, we see middle-class people just doing their things, but behind the front doors on Wisteria Lane, there's a story in each house. Well, every car from which you take a toll has an occupant with a different story. Make up the stories, figure out why the woman in the brand-new navy blue suit looked so tense as she drove through—

was she on her way to interview for a new job, was she worried that the suit wasn't sexy enough for the lover she was driving to meet? Smile and say to that woman, "You'll get the job," or "You look great" as she drives past your toll-booth. Doesn't matter if she heard or not. So, you can be a clerk at the super-market or a maid in a motel: if you breathe insight into your job, it's no longer boring. Maybe you will write the novel.

You know what? You've got it going on, right now, just as you are. I feel that. Be good to yourself, believe you're worthy and beautiful inside and out. Do something about your weaknesses that really do exist. Get the teeth fixed; if you feel dumb, take a course and become an expert in something; take a makeup lesson if you don't know how to use blusher. But listen: if you're able to get up every morning and stand on two legs in that toll-taker or supermarket uni-form, and meet and greet new people, you are worthy, you are blessed, you can make of the day what you want it to be. Believing that should raise your self-esteem, child.

And now that you like yourself better, you'll also have no trouble making friends. I'm totally crazy about my friends, but I've learned to be careful where in my life I put them. Read on.

Friendship

Be courteous to all but intimate with few, and let those few
be well tried before you give them your confidence.

GEORGE WASHINGTON

I was always very organized, very specific when it came to my career—I thought it all out magnificently. But I didn't approach my emotional life in the same way I did my professional life. In fact, I was plain old sloppy when it came to being the best I could be. Whatever anyone wanted, I gave. Whatever any strong per-son thought, I tried to think the same way. I didn't assess my strengths or my weaknesses—I trusted to luck. I never protected myself from bad influences because I expected everyone to love and protect me. And not everyone did.

The first thing I had to do to make myself strong was to surround myself with health-giving, positive people, the human forces in my life that would make me feel secure. That meant I had to limit the spaces around me—limit the access the world had in my life.

Then, a miracle: one day, when I was feeling drained, my pastor gave me the great gift of an image that showed me how to do it, made it all shining clear. I share that image with you.

"Think of yourself as a dartboard," Pastor A. R. Bernard said. "You're the center of that board—and if you remember what a dartboard looks like, the center is the tiniest circle. It's the center that everyone tries to reach. When you hit it, you get the greatest number of points. That center circle doesn't hold much space. If too many people converge on that tiniest circle, it becomes obliterated.

"Notice," continued the pastor, "that the concentric circles all get larger as they get away from the center. There's plenty of room in *those* circles."

Absolute

When you bring people into the spaces in your life, you give them access; and when you give access, you open your heart and become vulnerable.

I understood what Pastor Bernard was trying to tell me. My friends, family, colleagues, and acquaintances should have their special places in the circles around me: that was the best way to ensure my emotional well-being. I was allowing everyone into the smallest circle nearest me—I wasn't being selective. And it was driving me nuts. Different people advised me differently. Everyone wanted different things from me. I was being pulled in a million directions, and I was being agreeable, giving and giving—even when it wasn't in my best interests. I was letting people into circles that, frankly, they hadn't earned. Maybe that sounds a little snobby to you; I can't help it. It's true. I learned that people do have to earn their way into your trust and your heart. It's not that I'm a snob—

I promise you that—I'd never allow myself to be a snob! But it's of utmost importance to protect yourself when you're getting your emotional house in order.

I'll give you an example: some people want you to stay put where it's most comfortable for them. It's not that they're mean or nasty, just that they're accustomed to you being one kind of person—and even if it's not right for you, they encourage you to stay put. When I was fat and alone, there were many in my inner circle who were okay with Star = Fat and Alone. They could never see me being physically fit and trim and with someone. They weren't protecting me from bad health or low self-esteem; they never thought about encouraging me to be the best I could be. They really didn't belong in my inner circle.

Only one thing to do: I rearranged my circles.

In that tiny, inner circle today live my parents; my sister, Sheila; and my two dearest friends, Vanessa Bell Calloway and Janet Rollé. And unless you live on a distant planet, you know that when I was ready for love, I finally did meet the man of my dreams, Al Reynolds. Of course, he also lives in that tiny circle closest to me. I also added his mother Ms. Ada to this circle. Her prayers have literally saved my sanity. That circle is like my second skin. I know that when it all comes down, these people have my best interest at heart. They will always be my rocks of emotional and mental stability—I can trust them. They always have my back.

In the next circle are some real good friends—my "big sisters," Aunt Van, Judy, Blaine, Gwen, Dale, and LaTanya; Al's brother Ed and his wife Pam; and of course the Angels who watch over me, my bridesmaids: Lela, Lita, Holly, Cheryl, Vivica, Natalie, Marva, Denise, Lisa, Tara, Dette, Karenna—they're all there, they're my girls, I love them, I depend on them, and they depend on me, I wouldn't trade them for the world. This circle is also precious. But by the same token, I have learned that I need to take care of myself, make the decisions best for me, be dominated psychologically by no one person, be in thrall to no one person. Everyone needs to be her own best advocate. That's emotional strength. So, I keep some space between me and that second circle—even though my love always lives there.

In the other circles of that dartboard live other family members, my "boys," my other girlfriends (the "Hostesses"), friends, colleagues, and role models. They're all vitally important to my life, they're amusing, interesting, helpful, and very much a part of my life—but I now know, they're not *first-circle impor-tant.* In my life, they're in their correct place. When you're getting yourself in mental shape, you've got to be clear about priorities. You've got to keep people where they belong—and that's not always closest to your heart and trust.

Arrange your circles.

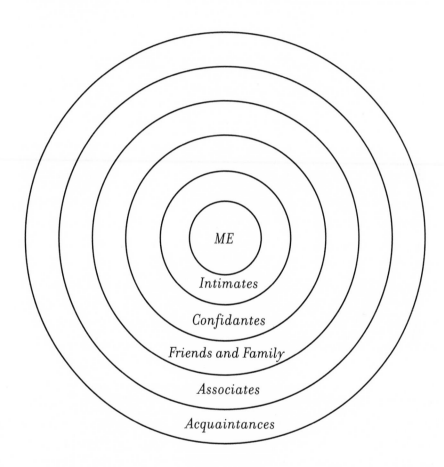

How to Arrange Your Circles

On a sheet of paper, draw your dartboard with six circles that get increasingly larger. Label the smallest center circle in the dartboard, Me. Label the next smallest circle and each of the rest as the circles get bigger:

Intimates

Confidantes

Friends

Associates

Acquaintances

On the bottom of the paper, answer the following questions in order, and place the names you come up with in the proper circles.

Note: I've used the female gender to make this exercise simpler, but every she or her could be a he or him—depending on who's on your list.

First circle: Me.

Second circle: These are your Intimates—the few people who are like a second skin to you. Here are the questions to ask yourself as you place people in this tiny, inner circle:

• Whom do you love and who loves you unconditionally?

• If you lost everything you had in a hurricane, who would drive to the border of your state, wait sixteen hours until you got there, then take you to her home for as long as you needed to stay?

• About whom, after she shares something, do you never have to ask, "Well, I wonder what's her real motivation in sharing that?"

• Whom would you trust to raise your children if something happened to you?

Third circle: These are your Confidantes—your beloved friends. These are the questions you should ask yourself to determine who fits in this circle:

• Whom do you trust with your secrets?

• Whom do you turn to in time of trouble?

• Whom do you immediately think of when you say "best friend"?

Fourth circle: Your Friends and Family. These are people you love and like enormously—they are close to you and you feel close to them. Ask the following questions of yourself to see who belongs in this circle:

• Whose wedding wouldn't you miss?

• Whose birthday do you never forget, and who never forgets yours?

• Who do you refer to as your "sister," "cousin," or "Aunt" when they really aren't . . . but really are?

• With whom do you shop and vacation?

Fifth circle: Your Associates. These are admired people you usually feel fondness for in your business and personal life.

• Who stays late at work with you when the pressure's on, shows up on time when she's supposed to be somewhere, and gossips with you when you need that?

• Whom do you rely on to test new ideas?

• Who are you glad to see at events?

• Who do you mutually promise you'll call socially—but rarely do?

Sixth circle: Your Acquaintances. This is the largest circle of people in your life. Some you wish you knew better; some you vaguely distrust but need; some you just think are interesting. You have to ask yourself only one question to see who belongs in this circle:

• Be honest whom do you often like, sometimes need, but really wouldn't miss for a minute if you never saw her again as long as you live?

Take this chart, analyze it, fill it out, evaluate it, and live it. You've finally put people where they belong in your life. Now treat them accordingly.

Chapter 5

Think Like a Lawyer

When you're getting yourself emotionally ready, in the way you *feel* about your self-esteem, your friendships, or your finances, it's also very helpful to change the way you *think* about all this. The way you mentally analyze your relationships and why you act the way you do is of paramount importance. We've learned that you can make changes in the way you feel, but can you actually change the way you think and act so that friendships and finances and true love arrive in a more intelligently planned way? Well, yes—I do believe you can reconstitute your thought processes. One of the reasons I so love being a lawyer is because lawyering, in a direct way, led me to my best life with my best partner, Al. It wasn't even the lawyering by itself that helped me change my life—it was the lawyer-think. Lawyers just think about things differently from most other people.

Absolute

How to make decisions: think, feel, then act.
If you feel, and then think, you are reasoning
based on your emotions and acting accordingly.

Okay, let's get them out of the way—the lawyer jokes:

Q. How does a pregnant woman know she's carrying a future lawyer?
A. She has an extreme craving for baloney.

Q. And God said, "Let there be Satan, so people don't blame everything on me . . .
A. And let there be lawyers, so people don't blame everything on Satan."

Q. Why won't sharks attack lawyers?
A. Professional courtesy.

Say what you will, lawyers are a pretty clever group as a whole. First of all, they're rarely boring. Second of all, they ponder stuff, they plan creatively, they have to convince others of the justness and rightness of their side. They're good at what they call *discovery*—finding out facts and evidence that will lead them to the best results.

So, the lawyer jokes may be funny, but they don't tell the whole story about the profession because the one thing lawyers do best is think things out. The paradox is that I could do that wonderfully well in the courtroom, but somehow the skill eluded me when I was just being Star.

I decided to try to carry the kind of thinking I did for my professional life into my personal life. I was convinced that would be the best emotional and mental preparation I could find.

You know what? I believe that everyone—every doctor, plumber, painter, mother, Home Depot salesperson—ought to think like a lawyer. Honestly, I'm not prejudiced because I'm a lawyer; a lot of my colleagues underwhelm me. It's just that thinking like a good lawyer makes your route to emotional preparedness very clear and simple. Hear me out.

If you want to make your case and win it, if you want to figure things out so they work to your advantage, if you want to clearly see both sides of a problem—and then make a sound decision—think like a lawyer. Whether you're contemplating a job change, throwing a not-terrific boyfriend out on his ear, making or terminating a friendship—think like the best lawyer I ever met, Johnnie Cochran Jr. When I wanted to find love, I thought, "What would Johnnie do?"

I was a long time coming to this "think like a lawyer" concept. I've told you that I did not approach my emotional life in the same way I approached my professional life. A lot of professional women make the same error. In deciding to be a nurse, teacher, accountant, or lawyer, the successful people are usually very methodical about how they plan it. They know how many years of school it will take, the organizations they need to join, how they want to look when they come to work. But when it comes to their inner emotional preparedness, they're often messes.

Believe me, I was one of those people. I joined Alpha Kappa Alpha sorority in college because it's the oldest black women's social service organization in the country, and I knew, wherever I moved, there would be a group of professional, college-educated women in Alpha Kappa Alpha with whom I could affiliate; they would be a built-in group of friends wherever I moved, and in Washington, DC; New York City; Houston, Texas; Los Angeles, California, I *have* established an easy and helpful relationship with these sorority sisters. I was methodical. I chose a law school based on how quickly its graduates passed the bar because I wanted to have a leg up in passing that exam, first time around. I was methodical. I interviewed and was offered jobs at several district attorney's offices around the country, but I chose the Brooklyn DA because I did my homework and learned that that office moved people along in their careers very quickly. I was methodical.

When I came to work on *The View*, I found it very difficult to have a conversation that didn't bring in my legal training because it was so useful in coming to the right decision. Sometimes, I guess it gets on people's nerves, but be sure I'll throw in an "allegedly" every little once in a while just to keep my legal edge.

But in my personal life, all these smarts flew out the window. I was haphazard, I was all over the place, I constantly made the same bad choices with men. I did not think like a lawyer. I was the antithesis of methodical.

But as I began to systematically prepare myself for love, it came to me that there was no better way to do it than by using the tried-and-true elements of legal thinking—the elements of a trial. I could make a better case for my personal future if I knew how to find evidence, look at the exhibits—build a case, period.

Follow me, step by step, and when you're preparing yourself for a relationship, when you're truly ready for love, you'll be a winner if you think like a lawyer getting ready for trial.

The Elements of a Trial
(And Finding and Building a Relationship)

A. Jury Selection: Your Peers Will Judge You

In any trial, the law requires a jury of your peers. In your personal life, it's the same thing. You need to look closely at your peer group. Who are the people who will judge you? Who are the people you must judge? Try to select a jury of your peers; those are the people with whom you should hang out.

I have a friend who's a brilliant neurosurgeon, Dr. Keith Black; he's also African American, one of the most gifted medical men in our country and we are both involved in an effort for brain cancer research in honor of his patient and our friend, the late Johnnie Cochran. "When you're choosing your friends," I once heard Keith say, "I think it's important to choose a group of friends who are achieving more than you are. That's the peer group you want, that's the jury of your peers. If you choose a group of friends who are achieving less, your friends will want to keep you in their group, they will continue to bring you down. The group of friends who achieve more will attempt to bring you up so you'll be part of their group."

That thought resonated with me.

When you're getting ready to form a relationship, do the same thing. You want to affiliate with a group that's going to give you the opportunity to meet the partner you need, the person with whom you want to talk—and talk, and then talk some more. If politics is important to you, hang with an achieving group who have similar political backgrounds. Volunteer to work in their organizations. They will judge you well.

If religion is important to you, find the purest, smartest, most appealing religious group on the planet—and join it. You will find men and women there whom you judge highly.

One of my matrons of honor, Janet, loves tennis. She serves on one of the committees of the United States Tennis Association, and her husband, Mark, was an amateur tennis player in college and very well ranked. Today, when they sit down together to watch Wimbledon or the French Open, they share their mutual delight in the sport. She didn't hang with a group of people just because they were friendly to her, she actively selected, she chose a jury of her peers to hang with—and the sunshine in her life was on that jury.

Now, be clear: I'm not talking about wealth, even though your mom might have said if you want to marry a rich man, don't hang out with a poor guy. You can be wealthy in knowledge, experience, education, social life, as well as dollars—it depends on what you value. Hang out with that jury.

I remember reading in the Old Testament that you don't want to be *unequally yoked*—you don't want to be with someone who can't pull his side of the wagon, doesn't share your core values, your interests. Opposites may attract, but they don't often last forever, which is why you should always marry a guy with whom you can be equally yoked. Remember the friend I mentioned, the neurosurgeon Dr. Keith Black? He recently told me that when he went looking for a mate, he too had a list. He wanted someone intelligent, goal-oriented, worldly, athletic, and pretty. He also wanted someone a daughter could use as a role model for the woman she would one day become. Well, he hit the jackpot. His wife, Dr. Carol Bennett, is a urologist who fills his list and more—that woman has it going on. Dr. Black sought someone who would complement and challenge his mind, body, and soul. Shouldn't you? When you purposefully try to associate with a jury of your peers, you'll meet people whose values and absolutes mesh with yours, whose life pursuits you judge highly. You will make relationships that do last forever.

B. The Opening Statement: First Impressions

The next stage of a trial is the opening statement, where you present and represent your case. As you do this, first impressions are crucial. For example, no intelligent lawyer goes into court badly or loudly dressed. She works hard not to offend the jury. Almost surely, she won't wear garish clothing or snagged pantyhose. When you appear at any job on the first day, you've purposely picked out appropriate clothing. If you work in a dance hall, you'll wear flashy stuff. If you work in an office, you'll be dressed down.

Think of dress as costume; it enhances the part you play.

When you go out on a date and you're looking for that special person, are you going to be someone who uses foul language? Are you appropriately dressed but sloppy (bra strap showing, shoes scuffed)? Do your dark roots show in your blond hair?

First impressions include being knowledgeable about the world. I watch *60 Minutes* every Sunday. It's "appointment" television for me because when I was a young girl, my family would always have an appointment on Sunday nights to gather and watch it and then have a discussion on one of the three issues presented. When you go out with a new guy, what have you got to offer in conversation? How will you maneuver the date into an experience he can't forget?

You are your own opening statement: how you look and how you act and sound is your brochure. Remember: there are people observing us from the sidelines at all times. If you're wearing a shirt cut down to your navel, swigging beer, and talking loudly and crudely, forget about attracting the young architect from Harvard or the successful businessman: your opening statement is awful. Well, maybe you'll attract him for a quickie relationship (I use the term lightly), but a booty call is not what you really want, is it?

Remember—you can always change your opening statement if it's not working well for you. But the first thing you can do is make an assessment of who you are today, who you want to become tomorrow—and dress, act, and sound the part.

C. The Case in Chief: Offer Your Best Evidence

The case in chief is the direct evidence you will present to the jury. It goes deeper than the opening statement. A trial lawyer very carefully prepares this evidence. And you must do the same. The best way to do it is to take a long, hard look at what you've become, whom you've chosen as friends, and where you spend your time. If you're satisfied with what you see as you assess yourself, fine—keep it just that way. If not, you can choose to make changes. The worst thing to do is to accept ambiguity—to agree with everybody and all the choices you've made in the past. No good lawyer agrees with everybody.

So, question your past and your present, question your evidence the way a two-year-old would. Ask why, just like a two-year-old: *why* did I go out with him, *why* am I spending so much time with friends who bore me, *why* aren't I doing something to perk up my mind? Every rule of law has a reason for its existence, and if you see something in your personality or habits that you automatically do without a good reason, question it and change it.

Absolute

∾

Be careful of what you love,
because whatever you love you will make a part of your life.

Here's a great way to question things. Write yourself down on paper.

In real life, if I wrote me up on paper (and I was scrupulously truthful), what evidence would others read? What would my case in chief look like?

When I really began to deal with my personal life (and not a trial), I started to keep a seven-day journal. This became my case in chief, the direct evidence of my lifestyle. It helped me step back and look at myself closely—and be pleased or displeased. The evidence gave me a clear look at the way my life had been going. I got the idea when I started my weight-loss program and my nutritionist told me to keep a food journal. How could I figure out what to eat if I didn't already know what I'd been eating—and believe me, you forget unless you write it down. The food journal would be evidence of what I'd consumed that week.

So, I decided to keep a seven-day personal journal for evidence of the lifestyle I was leading. For the first time really, I began to think like a lawyer in my personal life. I made many objections to what I saw as I reread it. My case in chief was weak. My evidence about myself was incriminating. And so, I consciously began to change the way I made decisions about men, friends, and my lifestyle in general.

I suggest you try it. Check out your calendar, Palm Pilot, or BlackBerry for help in remembering your week. And start writing down, for seven days, most of everything you do and think and everybody you see.

Question yourself and answer the questions. Of course, you can make up your own questions that best reveal your evidence, but here were mine:

* *Where have I been this week?* Write down every single place. Are you happy with where you have gone? Could you have gone to more productive, interesting places? Like what? Be specific!
* *With whom have I hung out?* Name every single person. Are they a jury of your peers?
* *What were my impressions of those people, those places?* Did they change you for the better? For the worse? How? Be specific!
* *What restaurants have I visited?* Have you eaten with respect for your body—or scarfed down just anything?
* *What movies or shows have I seen?* How have they informed your thinking?
* *What books or magazines have I read?* How have they informed your thinking?
* *What activities or sports have I played?* Have they made you feel physically fit?

❋ *With what man (men) have I been even a little intimate?* Happy with yourself?

❋ *With whom have I argued?* Was it worth it?

❋ *To whom did I lie?* Are you glad or sorry you lied?

❋ *With whom have I felt safe and inspired?* Is he or she a regular in your life? Why not?

❋ *Has there been a single person or act during this week that made me change my life for the better?* How does that make you feel?

❋ *What has made me frustrated—or ashamed of myself?* (Name as many things as are true.)

❋ *What has made me proud or satisfied with myself?* (Name as many things as are true.)

❋ *What did I thank God for, and what did I pray for?* Be specific.

❋ Finally, taking your journal beyond seven days, *how many relationship failures in the last year or so have I noticed?* Why have they failed—his fault or partly yours?

When the seven days are over, check out your diary. Do you see places where you have to make changes? Are you happy and proud with how your case in chief, the case for yourself, is shaping up?

I recently looked back in my Palm Pilot to remember what I did the week I met Al, and I was proud. I traveled to South Carolina for *The View*, attended two charity events, played poker with Whoopi, and exercised four times that week. I met Al on a night when I was happy, healthy, and apparently ready for love. Looking back now, two years later, the week still looks good on paper.

If your case in chief doesn't look good on paper, Kendra, it's probably worse in reality.

D. The Rebuttal Case: Where Are the Weaknesses of Your Case? How Can You Overcome Those Weaknesses?

If you're really thinking like a lawyer, you'll put on a rebuttal case. That's the time to cross-examine and make objections to your case in chief. That's the time to see how many red flags in your life have been raised—flags that have been shouting, *Caution! Not Good! Don't Go There! Oh God, I Went There and It's Such a Drag!* And that's the time to make objections and corrections to your actions, if necessary. Were those red flags there because of something you yourself did or didn't do—or were they truly someone else's fault? Now ask yourself the toughest question:

How many of my relationship failures are not really because he did me wrong, but because I shouldn't have chosen that person in the first place?

If your answer is that he really did you wrong, and you made no false judgments in choosing him, and your life is praiseworthy and happy, you have no rebuttal case. But if you cross-examine yourself and see that it was you who was mostly responsible for the failures, you are doing yourself some real good by this candid self-assessment, this personal rebuttal.

Let me be honest. Every time I was in a relationship before I met my husband, a shrill bell went off pretty early—and I ignored it. I should have listened to the bell and walked away.

Absolute

*Although we have the capacity to know,
we can be conditioned to ignore.*

That bell ringing should have led me to a powerful rebuttal case. For example, one relationship failed because of my overwhelming desire to be nurturing—even though I was getting no nurturing back: this man had a mother, so I didn't need to nurture him. Another poor relationship failed because I thought I could fix what was wrong about him—and you all know that can never happen: grown people are what they are, they're not ever changing, you take 'em as you get 'em.

Another happened because I didn't want to be alone and I settled for less than what I deserved. I didn't realize that being alone should not be the same as being lonely. I had to find other activities that made me happy. A friend of mine had low self-esteem, so she committed to the first wrong guy she met. She didn't think she was worthy of anyone better than the guy in her life. Another friend found herself in an abusive relationship and didn't know how to get out, so she stayed. What rebuttal cases they made.

Do you see yourself in one of those situations? Be discerning, be truthful, so the next time they occur, you'll hear that shrill bell. We tell our kids that when a strange man or woman comes up to them and gives them that uh-oh feeling, they should turn on their heels and run. If you see your boyfriend's (or even your own) behavior in a relationship that's giving you an uh-oh feeling, *run*. That's the best rebuttal.

E. The Witnesses: Who's Testifying for You, Child?

Your case is really only as good as your witnesses. Your witnesses are the people who know the facts about you—they are your intimates, your friends, acquaintances, and associates—and they will testify to what they have seen or heard about you. They're different from a jury, which, only after having seen and heard the witnesses (your evidence), decides where the truth lies. When you're preparing your rebuttal case, know that the other side will look at your witnesses: your girlfriends and male friends tell an awful lot of truth about you. Whom have you chosen to spend time with, and why? Believe me, you will be judged by your witnesses.

But, remember, we're still dealing with a rebuttal case here. When you meet someone, you must also think, Who are *his* witnesses? That was a big, big deal for me. Thinking like a lawyer, I knew I would be able to tell so much about a guy by the people in his life.

So, when I met Al, I knew I should look at his witnesses. His friends and family, I soon found out, were the salt of the earth. I would be with a jury of my peers in his group, because like me, he came from a small Southern town. His family had been public and social servants of their communities—his mom was an educator, his father had been in the military, and all five siblings were college graduates. Sounded good. He also told me he'd been looking for someone he'd be proud to bring to his witnesses, his own family.

But thinking like a lawyer and looking closely, I also saw what could be problems for me in this relationship. I saw how funny he was with his mom and aunts: how they idolized him and interacted with him as their center could make them a hard act to follow. I also noticed that he was spoiled and babied beyond belief by these women. His witnesses were telling me he'd require major babying and spoiling. Hmmm. Could I do it? I saw all that in a month, and he saw me clearly too in that month through my own family. Saw my ultra strength and my ultra bossiness. Hmmm. Could he deal with it?

I met his best buddies, his work colleagues; I went to his business Christmas party. I watched him help one friend move out of his apartment, and I thought, "Good—a giving person." I went to his church, and he came to mine because we were both interested in meeting each other's spiritual leaders. I watched him interact with his brothers and sisters. I saw who he was and who he always would be (guys don't change, Vanda). Then, second in significance only to my meeting his parents, I wanted to meet some of his female friends—not girls he dated, his girl *friends.* These witnesses, unconsciously, would tell me a lot about the man. They'd be very telling witnesses.

All his girls, Tamara, Lauren, Tamika, and Karen, were smart, capable, and gorgeous; they cared about him and wanted to make sure I wasn't a flake. They were, thank goodness, not hostile witnesses, but they would have turned hostile (baby, I felt it) if I was not worthy of their friend. I heard them say to him variations of "You better not hurt her." I also heard said to me, "You better not hurt him." It was important to hear all of it.

If the person you're interested in doesn't have a good relationship with his family and with friends who vouch for him and his character, then his witnesses just don't add up. The evidence, the exhibits are all there.

I was a tiny bit concerned about one thing, something basic in our characters—the different way we approached people. I approach life presuming people are good and honest and trustworthy. Maybe it's my legal training—the presumption of innocence stuff—but I do give everyone the benefit of the doubt. Instead of walling off or closing down, as many people in the public eye do, I am very welcoming.

This means what? It means I often end up disappointed.

> ## *Absolute*
>
> *Disappointment is not based on what you find,*
> *but on what you* expect *to find.*

Al, on the other hand, lives his life presuming you're going to screw him. He's sure that people aren't always on the up and up, and he deals with them accordingly.

This means what? It means he often ends up being pleasantly surprised. At the end of the day, I'm disappointed and he's pleasantly surprised. It's a big difference in outlook. Could we live with it—or would we drive each other nuts?

When I spoke to my pastor, he helped. He suggested that even when I was disappointed in the way people treated me, "the Bible says no weapon formed against you shall prosper. That doesn't mean, Star," he said, "that no weapon will be formed against you. There always will be people who hurt and disappoint you. It only means that, in the end, no weapon held against you will *prosper.* In the long run, the weapons of mean-spirited people will not work."

I could live with that, just as any Buddhist who is a good person with excellent karma mustn't believe that no one will ever hurt him again. He will be hurt again, but his enemies' weapons would not *prosper.*

And I could learn a little caution from my new husband-to-be. And maybe, he could learn to give *some* people the benefit of the doubt.

Al was a keeper.

F. The Summation: Assess Your Case and Sell It to the Jury

The lawyer's final job in presenting a case is the summation.

When you sum up, you must do a real assessment. Summation is the time when a person, thinking like a lawyer, does an evaluation of her case and blends it all together for the jury. You tie up your evidence, the other side's evidence, the witnesses' statements, you apply the law—and then you use your skill and talent to convince the jury that your side is the better side.

My pastor recently said something that truly touched my spirit.

It's very difficult for people in summarizing their lives, he said, not to be concerned with how people perceive them. And if you're in the public eye, as I am, it's even more difficult: we sit there every weekday, millions of people watch us on television, and our livelihoods and reputations all do rest on how others perceive us. But they don't really see our character. Our character doesn't depend on others' peripheral perceptions. On this day, my pastor gave a sermon in which he told us that it's far more important to be concerned with your character than with your reputation—far more important because we truly live in our characters, not in our reputations.

I believe that with all my heart.

Absolute

*If you worry about your reputation,
you will compromise your integrity.
Worry about your character.*

Back to summing up: only you can sum up, only you can assess your case—I can't do it for you. I don't know you. Only you really know you. And only you know the state of your character.

Look—when I did a summation on myself, I clearly saw some of my flaws. I'm bossy. I'm extremely controlling. I find it easier to do things myself rather than share in the doing. I've been working by myself for so long as an independent person, being part of a marital team would be difficult for me. That's who I am. I either had to do an honest evaluation of myself and have a desire to soften the elements that might rub a husband the wrong way—or recognize that whomever I was with had to be able to deal with those elements.

Al also had to do his own summing up. He was not a guy who was going to play second fiddle to me. If I wanted someone who would carry my bags through life, it wasn't going to be Al. About that bossiness part:

Today, quite often, Al says to me when I apologize for my overkill, "You're never *not* going to be controlling, Star, and I knew that when we were dating. I figured that I couldn't get freaked out every time you pulled that because that's who you are and I couldn't change you."

He was right. You can never change another person, but if you're convinced that something in your character is not good, you *can* change yourself. You can either recognize that the not-good stuff will be a grave impediment in your relationship, or at least try to soften the effect of the bad junk—even if you can't erase it completely.

So, here's the deal. When you meet a man who looks very wonderful and promising, you both need to think like lawyers. Sum up. Each of you make lists—what's the good stuff about yourself, what's the bad? Deal with your own bad junk before the other side deals with it—that's what lawyers do. Deal with the stuff that doesn't make your case look good. And deal with it actively. When you see the weakness in your case, try to minimize it. If you're in bad shape physically, make every effort to get healthy. If you're the kind of person who's nasty to others, try to soften it or fix it. Highlight the good stuff, and try to diminish the bad stuff by explaining to the other what it all means—that's where communication comes in.

Personally, let me be honest: when I started to look at what stood in my way, I was tunnel-visioned, like a horse with blinders. But then, when I did a real self-evaluation on myself, I want to be clear—I didn't fix everything that was weak. I figured that Al and I had to accept that certain parts were not ever going to totally change. I had to deliberate, look deep into the heart of my beloved to see if he could deal with me. He's a tough guy. He could.

But then, I also learned to compromise. Bend in the wind, like bamboo. And I think I did get somewhat more flexible. Maybe I'm not quite as bossy or controlling as I used to be—at least not with Al. But this you'd have to ask him yourself.

G. The Verdict: Is It Fair? Is It Just? Are You Satisfied with It?

Again—I can't help you here. Each of us has to come to her own verdict. Others will give you their assessment of your relationship or the problems at hand or whatever else you're working on, but your judgment on yourself should be the toughest and truest.

I want to say, if you have an ordered mind and you've prepared yourself for an honest decision, your verdict will be the correct one for you. Should you take the job, marry him, trust the new girlfriend, defy your boss? Deep in your heart, you know the right verdict.

By the Way—It's Okay to Dismiss Your Case

Here's a thought: you can back out of your case. If it looks shaky or snarky, if it gives you that uh-oh feeling, you don't have to carry through. You don't have to marry the guy, change your job, write the book, run for the presidency, drop a friend, if you see during summation that your case stinks.

I remember preparing to try a murder case when strong evidence came to light that the defendant was not the murderer. I had to be courageous enough to investigate the new evidence and then toss aside my carefully prepared case because even though there was a murder victim, even though I might not ever get the actual murderer, I had to be honest with myself and face the fact that the guy I had was not the guy I wanted.

So, if you meet a man and all the evidence and all the witnesses say the guy you have is not the guy you wanted, he's not your guy. Dismiss the case. Move on. You'll get rid of him before you get hurt, before you even wait for a complete verdict. If you are thinking about changing your job and after you investigate a new job the way a lawyer would, and you find out the new job will probably be more onerous than the present one, dismiss the case. Move on. If you hear that your best friend has said awful things about you, and you investigate it—and determine that it's probably just a vicious, untrue rumor, dismiss the case, hug your friend, and move on.

Think like a lawyer.

Chapter 6

Getting Your Financial House in Order

The lack of money is the root of all evil.

GEORGE BERNARD SHAW

I have enough money to last me the rest of my life unless I buy something.

JACKIE MASON

It is better to have a permanent income than to be fascinating.

OSCAR WILDE

What do your finances have to do with getting yourself emotionally ready to find love? If you have to ask, you really need this chapter. It's no secret that money is the number one cause of arguments in a marriage. Even the happiest couples occasionally fight or, at best, feel very cranky about the way their partners handle (or don't handle) the family funds. In essence, finances drive emotions, and if you have babyish, immature responses to managing money, trust Auntie Star—there's trouble ahead.

You can be seventy-two and still be a babe in the woods about money smarts. There's no question in my mind that one of the most important things you can do to get ready to meet That Guy is have your financial house in order. I mean, sure, you can meet a terrific man even if your finances are a mess, but marrying him and keeping him is another story—not the story I want to tell, not even the story I want to read.

Even if you never end up married (and deep down, I won't believe that's going to happen if you're ready for marriage), for your own happiness and well-being, you've just got to be financially healthy and independent. I mean, girl—here we are in the twenty-first century. Jane Austen no longer rules. Your own financially secure name is your ticket to safety. And make no mistake, earning a lot of money is swell, but the ability to make practical goals, practical investments, practical decisions, *and* live within your income is really the name of the game.

Before we begin, assess yourself today. Take the following quiz to see how savvy and sophisticated you are about money.

HOW GROWN-UP ARE YOU ABOUT MONEY?

PART I: Answer true or false to the following statements (and lying is really not allowed).

1. I read my monthly investment and/or bank statements carefully.	TRUE	FALSE
2. I have a *written* financial life plan, a goal toward which I am working.	TRUE	FALSE
3. I often make purchases that I later regret.	TRUE	FALSE

4. I know what a mutual fund and a REIT are.	TRUE	FALSE
5. I keep records of my income and deductions as the IRS requests (only until the end of the next tax year).	TRUE	FALSE
6. I own my own home.	TRUE	FALSE
7. I have never attended a financial seminar or workshop: What am I, a banker?	TRUE	FALSE
8. I've never invested in stocks or bonds. I trust only my savings account.	TRUE	FALSE
9. I have more than twenty credit cards: I spread my debt around.	TRUE	FALSE
10. I can't afford an education. No worry, I'm bright and determined, and I'll make it on my street smarts.	TRUE	FALSE

Part II: NOW CHOOSE THE BEST ANSWER TO THE FOLLOWING QUESTIONS (Again, tell the truth, girlfriend—don't choose the answer you think I want to hear.)

11. You're short of money, but you need a fabulous, very expensive new dress you've seen. You:

A. Buy it. You said "need," didn't you?
B. Go to an outlet and see if you can find a similar one, cheaper
C. Wait till it goes on sale
D. Walk away

12. My checkbook is almost always:

A. Not filled out with dates or amounts (I fill it in later, when I have time)
B. Confusing, but I usually can figure it out
C. Lost
D. Balanced

continued

13. The best way to get a good credit rating is to:

A. Borrow money
B. Give excellent personal references
C. Dress fashionably and give a cheery smile to bankers
D. Sign a pledge of morality

14. You feel you have an unexplored talent—maybe to be a lawyer, interior designer, or writer, you:

A. Feel cheated you weren't born rich so you could pursue your dream
B. Try really hard to do it on your own
C. Dream about it; plan to pursue it when you have more time and money
D. Take a course or go back to school for a degree—even if you have to borrow the money

15. When was the last time a creditor bothered you about an unpaid bill?

A. How about yesterday? Maybe an hour ago?
B. Within the month
C. I can't remember
D. Never

16. I seek financial advice from:

A. Almost everyone—I'm always open to hearing other opinions
B. Only friends and relatives who care about me and want nothing from me
C. Colleagues or bosses
D. Competent professionals

17. I save:

A. When I feel rich
B. When I worry there's going to be financial trouble ahead
C. Part of every paycheck
D. When I remember—that's pretty often

18. My credit cards are:

A. In my name
B. In the name of my workplace—I have an expense account to use
C. I don't have credit cards: it's wiser to avoid temptation
D. In the name of my parents or husband: it's easier for me that way

19. Regarding retirement plans at work:

A. I have a 401(k) but stopped contributing: I'm young, I want to live in the present, not the future, and I have barely enough to get along on now.

B. I contribute regularly but as little as I can: when I'm older, I'll raise my contribution.

C. I save on my own: I don't trust these business savings plans—what if they go bankrupt?

D. I contribute as much as I can.

E. I don't have a job that offers retirement plans.

20. This is my real financial philosophy, even though I may not announce it:

A. "It's just as easy to marry a rich man as a poor man," say many mothers. I believe it. And men should be the primary providers in a family.

B. "We can tell our values by looking at our checkbook stubs." (Gloria Steinem)

C. "All good things come to those who wait." (I don't remember who said it.)

D. Move forward, take calculated risks, and invest well even if you can't afford it, right now.

E. Seize the moment. "Remember all those women on the *Titanic* who waved off the dessert cart." (Erma Bombeck)

Part III: The next five questions are geared to determine whether or not you have a "winner's mystique" (that is, a clear indication of your money maturity).

21. You appear to be making no impression at all at a business meeting. That's because:

A. Basically, you're a bubblehead trying to be adorable.

B. You haven't done your homework.

C. You're listening hard, rather than saying anything.

D. You're wearing gaucho pants.

22. You've had problems in the past with your credit. You want to start off with a clean slate with a new lending institution. It's a good idea:

A. Without actually lying, don't offer any information about your past credit problems.

B. Use another name—say, your mom's maiden name—with the lending institution.

C. Open a new bank account and a new charge account. Use them responsibly for a few months before applying to the new lending institution.

D. Understand that you can sue the new lending institution for turning you down before you do anything bad. Tell them you know about this law.

continued

23. Your finances haven't improved in two years. Why?

A. Not my fault. Others have cheated and edged me out unfairly.

B. I'm due for a raise in about a year.

C. So what? Money isn't everything. I'm making contacts.

D. So what? I've just gone out on my own in a new business.

24. You've just been offered a step up the corporate ladder. Your office space will remain the same.

A. Good—it's small but cozy and near your friends.

B. You think, "I couldn't care less where I sit—I'm thrilled to be promoted."

C. You understand that power and influence have nothing to do with where you sit.

D. You request that there be some change in your physical surroundings.

25. Your credit rating is greatly enhanced if you:

A. Pay for everything in cash.

B. Pay bills immediately after getting a late notice.

C. Use your credit card to buy stuff (even though you can afford the cash).

D. Pay your bills the minute you receive them.

E. Marry Bill Gates Jr.

ANSWERS

Part I

Take 50 points if you answered True to questions 1, 2, 3, and 6.

Take 50 points if you answered False to questions 5, 7, 8, 9, and 10.

Take 20 points if you got four or more correct.

If you got under four correct, take 0.

Just for your information, you should keep financial records for at least three years (and sometimes, as in the case of deeds, bonds, etc.) forever. Basically, a mutual fund is a type of investment that consists of a pool of investment, rather than a single stock; a REIT is a real estate investment. If you are at all involved in investing your funds, you should know the language. You'll find the other answers within the next few pages, but just one more thing for now: *no one* needs twenty credit cards.

Part II

11. If you answered <u>B,</u> take 10 points

12. If you answered <u>D,</u> take 10 points

13. If you answered **A**, take 10 points. If you answered **C** or **D**, subtract 10 points.

14. If you answered **D**, take 20 points

15. If you answered **D**, take 10 points

16. If you answered **D**, take 10 points

17. If you answered **C**, take 10 points

18. If you answered **A**, take 10 points

19. If you answered **D**, take 10 points

20. If you answered **D**, take 10 points. If you answered **A**, subtract 10 points.

Part III

21. If you answered **B**, take 10 points. If you answered the gaucho pants thing, subtract 20 points. Why would anyone wear gaucho pants to a business meeting?

22. If you answered **C**, take 10 points. If you answered **A** or **B**, subtract 10 points. Trying to fool the organization will get you not far at all.

23. If you answered **D**, take 10 points. It's the only answer that shows smarts.

24. If you answered **A**, take 10 points. Experts say that people who are satisfied to work in cubicles rarely make it to the top. A job promotion should also mean a larger office, or one with a view or a larger desk or *some* visible change in the place you sit: the message you then send is "I'm on the way up."

25. If you answered **C**, take ten points. If you answered **A**, subtract 10 points: paying in cash does zilch for your credit rating.

ANALYSIS

Add your points.

If you scored under 180
Yikes. You need help, momma. Your house is not in good financial order. Quick—get some money smarts. It's not difficult—I promise. Put down the sex chapter and read this one, first. Then, take a course.

continued

If you scored from 180 to 200
Not terrific but not the pits, either. You have the basics but you need to learn the fine points of protecting yourself in the real (money) world. You'll get along if you either get some professional advice or read this chapter twice.

If you scored from 210 to 230
Not too shabby a score, at all. You've obviously had some sophisticated experience dealing with money, and all you need is a refresher course. Read on.

If you scored from 240 to 260
If Bill Gates weren't married, he'd make a pitch for you—that's how moneywise you are. Congratulations. Read the following chapter anyway: I guarantee you'll find new tips on how to make yourself financially independent.

✳   ✳   ✳

There's Only One Chris Rock, and She's Got Him

So here's one of my favorite stories:

Chris Rock and his wife, Malaak, are two of my very dear friends. One day, Chris came on *The View,* and during the interview I asked him to tell me about the most romantic thing he'd ever done for his wife.

Chris's response? "I cleaned up her credit."

Everybody was laughing hard because he's a brilliant comedian, but guess what—I know Malaak, and she's so gifted and talented I'd bet my engagement ring he sure didn't need to clean up her credit.

But suppose he did? Let me break it to you gently: You all out there might not get a Chris Rock who can or who wants to clean up your credit.

You sit there and think to yourself, Ooh wouldn't I just love to have a man come in my life and wipe out my debts. Well, I have news for you: you won't. Unless you meet one of those guys who's in the credit cleanup business, you need to clean up your credit all by yourself because no man wants to come in and have to start fixing you. No one wants to start a relationship by taking on a financial burden—and further, you don't want to have to be dependent on a guy. Believe me—you *don't*. You want to be able to bring something to the table other than an appetite.

It's time-out for the old, unwise emotion of "I want a man to take care of my bills."

I'm not suggesting that a couple has to be financially equal. I could always handle someone I loved who came to me with a little baggage, and most good men would probably feel that way about a woman they loved. But, honey, I can just hear the man of your dreams saying, "Please don't come into my life with a matched set of luggage upon luggage carrying $40,000 worth of Manolo Blahnik shoes; don't come into my life with a rented apartment when you can't even come up with the down payment to buy the apartment. I got to worry about this loan you have? I got to worry about your car note? I don't need Louis Vuitton trunks coming into my life, here. That will bring such financial burdens into the relationship. Let's not start off on very unequal footing."

We all know you're not attractive if your teeth are stained, you're anorexic or obese, or your hair needs a serious washing. You're even less attractive if you have bad credit, if you overspend, and if you can't pay your own way if you had to. A huge part of preparing yourself for love is getting your financial house in order.

Case in point: I know so many people in the music industry who hang $250,000 diamond medallions around their necks—and they're still renting rather than owning apartments. What, *what, WHAT* are you thinking, I want to ask.

On our first New Year's together as husband and wife, Al and I sat on the beach in St. Bart's and began to write out a plan: Al called it our business plan for life. It would consist of the goals and expectations our family—the two of us—would work on that year.

To help you do the same, I want to introduce you to Al Reynolds, my husband, former Wall Street banker, and the man who knows more than anyone else in my life about financial security. Today, he's a financial management executive dedicated to extremely high-net-worth individuals, and he advises them on every aspect of their financial lives, from helping them buy their art and yachts, to personal security for couples and singles. He's a financial doctor, a financial therapist, and a financial wizard. Most important, he advises me (with a great team of other professionals) on my finances—you don't think I'd entrust my own money to less than the best, do you? As I said, the best. He's my expert on this subject.

So, I give this task to him: explain some of the tenets of a solid financial house to my readers. You're in good hands.

Finances 101, According to Al Scales Reynolds

From a very young age, I was always taught to have a plan, and that plan would serve as a road map to wherever I was going. It's been the theme of my life, and I always work more on that road map—the process—than the actual goal. For example, if you tell me you want to be a banker, I'll give you a short but good plan. It looks like this:

> A. You need to go to a great college and earn a great grade-point average.
> B. You need to graduate with a degree in finance and then go on to get two years of experience with a top-ten financial company.
> C. In order to work in a top firm on Wall Street as a banker, you now need to go back to school and get an MBA.
> Did all that? Now you're ready.

Every woman who hopes to be in a serious relationship one day ought to start with a road map. It will help her build wealth, protect it, organize it, spend it, save it, and share it wisely. If you're single, start the road map with some serious thought about finances while following the game plan below; if you're in a relationship, with your partner, indulge in the same kind of straight talk about money and goals.

The Road Maps

Take out three big sheets of paper: these will be morphed into your financial road maps. On the first sheet, write down . . .

Time frame: Next two to three years

1. **What's my goal?** Put a price tag on this goal. If you want to live in Paris for a year, buy a house, have your own business, or whatever—figure out approximately how much it will cost for the next two to three years. (I didn't say making this plan would be easy!) Do I want to have a job where I get a paycheck every Friday—or do I want to plan long-term for a career? Decide on a goal, a time frame, and figure out approximately how much it will cost to attain.

2. **What are my present expenses?** Put an approximate dollar figure on this: add up approximately what you spend for housing, entertainment, clothes, food, travel, medical expenses, insurance, paying off debts, gifts—whatever.

3. **How much money will I need to accomplish my goal?** Subtract number 2 from number 1, and add 20 percent for unexpected expenses, inflation, and prices that may rise. Your answer will approximate how much money you will need to meet your goal.

4. **How much do I earn a year, now?** Look hard at this figure. How much more money than you have now will you need to accomplish your goal?

5. **What do I expect to be earning in the next two to three years?** Jot this down.

6. **What will I hopefully own at the end of that time?** Be as detailed as you need to be.

7. **What will I have accomplished? Can I meet my goal?**

On the second sheet of paper, ask yourself the same questions as in the first time frame, only change the time frame to:

Time frame: Next four to seven years

Then, on the third sheet, asking the same questions, write:

Time frame: Next ten years plus . . .

It may take you several weeks to fill out these business plans, which cover at least the next ten years. Be realistic, and add a bit more to whatever your figures come out to be in each category (things always cost more). Your answers will be your road map.

Try to stick to the map as closely as possible. Of course, things will change—you can't predict everything, but now, at least, you have a road map. The following are some tips on how to get to where you're going.

An Ordered Financial House—*If You Are Single*

Finances play a huge role in relationships: no surprise that it's the number one cause for divorce in America. There are so many emotions, so much anxiety and guesswork surrounding finances that if you don't sit down to figure out a financial game plan by yourself before you have a serious partner, there's going to be trouble.

Before you put your financial house in order as a couple, it makes eminent sense to deal with it as a single, right now, even before there's a husband on the horizon. Get a handle on what works for you alone, and you'll have far better "couple" judgment later on. What follows are some of the basics. I suggest you have:

An Emergency Exit Plan

It's simple: every woman, rich or poor, ought to be in control of her own money. That offers her a sense of security right off the bat.

Even for starters, every woman should have an emergency exit plan. In most cities, for example, every building has an emergency exit or fire escape plan consisting of signage and fire extinguishers that will aid each occupant to get out of the building in case of disaster. Although a woman doesn't anticipate that her house is going to burn down or her relationship is going to end, just in case that happens, she needs an exit plan.

The emergency exit plan consists of these things:

1. **Establish credit.** Credit cards should always be in your own name, and *kept* in your own name even after you marry. Establishing a sound

credit identity is one of the best things you can do for your future husband.

2. **Get out of debt.** Getting your financial house in order isn't about maxing out your credit by overcharging on those cards; it is about paying down the debt as soon as possible. Of course, it's sometimes impossible to swing the whole balance, every month.

So, here's the trick to sensibly paying off credit cards: if you pay just the minimum your credit card asks for, you'll *never* get free of Mastercard. Instead, look at your bill, find out the finance charge for that month, and add the minimum payment to it—then, let that be your minimum. If you can afford it, pay at least twice the minimum. If you get a bonus or a raise or birthday presents in the form of cash, take that money and send it straight to the credit company. Face it: it's true that the average person making $30,000 to $50,000 a year uses her credit cards to live. It's particularly important for her to manage finance charges responsibly, manage the interest she pays, and certainly, manage the amount she charges on those cards.

3. **When you're desperate, get help.** Sometimes the debt seems just too big a mountain to climb. Think about asking for the services of a debt counselor. There are many nonprofit credit-counseling agencies created to help people climb out of onerous debts. They can get lenders to lower their rates, eliminate late fees, extend your payment terms, or settle for less on what you owe. Check out the Web site Myvsta.org.

Other good Web sites and telephone numbers:

CardWeb.com (800-344-7714). The Ram Research Company, for a small fee, will give you a list of banks offering credit cards with very low finance charges, low or no yearly fees, secured credit cards for a person who wants to rebuild her poor credit history, and other information.

National Foundation for Consumer Credit (www.nfcc.org). If you're having credit problems, this is a great Web site. The nonprofit foundation will act as a mediator between you and the creditor, and can often negotiate very comfortable settlements. The service may be free, but if not, it will not cost more than $50. The address is 8701 Georgia Avenue, Suite 601, Silver Spring, MD 20910.

Computer debt management. If you want to get your debt under control online, consider Quicken.com, which is a financial site dedicated to finding a way for you to get out of debt, and then plan your future finances—after you insert your financial information.

Credit bureaus. These bureaus know everything about your credit, and they issue credit reports on you to anyone who asks. If you apply for a loan, a credit grantor will surely check out your credit report to decide whether or not you're a good credit risk. You can call or write any of the bureaus to get a copy of your credit report and see what others will be reading about you (and what bad credit you may have to clean up). Some bureaus may charge you a fee. IMPORTANT: Credit bureaus often have the wrong information about you. You certainly will want to have that information erased from your record, which is another reason to check what they're sending out about you. These are the three major credit bureaus:

Equifax Credit Information Services (404-885-8000): For a copy of the report, write PO Box 740241, Atlanta, GA 30375-0241.

Experian (800-354-5368): For a copy of their report, write Experian National Consumer Assistance Center, PO Box 2002, 701 Experian Parkway, Allen, TX 75013.

Trans Union Corporation (800-888-4213): For a copy of their report, write 760 W. Sproul Rd., PO Box 390, Springfield, PA 19064.

Whatever you do, however you do it—get that financial house in order by eliminating major credit card debt. The man of your dreams may appear momentarily, and if he's not Chris Rock, and he takes a look at a debt-ridden woman (cute as she may be), he may think you're a bad risk.

When you've done so, you have a good start on your emergency exit plan.

Star's Favorite Financial Tip

*I*nvest in your own education and job training even if you temporarily have to go into debt.

I've said you should avoid credit card debt. Is my wife contradicting me? No. She's right-on. If there's anything you should go into debt for, it's your education. Star did just that, and it increased her earning power enormously. The happiest day of her life came when she paid off those college loans, but her fairy-tale life wouldn't have happened without that education. Your education and training are your biggest assets.

Consider a bank loan, consider borrowing against the equity you may have in your home, and certainly consider applying for financial aid, which you can pay off as your earning power increases. Investigate lending institutions, including your credit union, to discover good lending rates; a good Internet source for checking out interest rates on bank loans is www.bankrate.com.

4. **Save as much as you can.** Figure to save 15 percent of your income, at least. You'll be happy you did. Once you get in the habit of saving, it doesn't hurt a bit. I strongly advise that after you pay your bills, you should pay yourself. If you're an independent woman, and you have ten bills for the month, the eleventh bill should be your own. Translated, that means that you give yourself a present and put a portion of what's left into a savings account. It builds up.

5. **Invest carefully.** After a while, piggy banks just don't do it. Your emergency exit plan (not to mention your living plan) is absolutely dependent on interest-bearing savings or brokerage accounts you build up in your own name.

  • Invest in the market? Should you buy a mutual fund or an individual stock? (It's the mutual fund, every time!)

- Should you hit the bond market?
- Should you diversify or put all your eggs in one solid basket?
- Should you take or reinvest your dividends?

You've absolutely got to educate yourself in this field. There are dozens of books on the market and even more experts on television, in your own bank, and in print who only want to help you think your way through to financial solvency. Don't listen slavishly to any one source, but become familiar with all the possibilities.

6. **Need a specialist?** For not very much money, you can even hire a financial consultant, whose job it is to build your money through asset allocation, evaluating your risk tolerance, and devising an investment strategy. Such a person can do as much or as little as you like. Some pick out the actual investments and manage your funds daily. Others meet or talk with you periodically just to make sure you understand how your portfolio is doing. You don't have to be rich to hire a financial planner, but remember, a consultant who gets paid a percentage on the growing amount of your portfolio is a better deal than one who is paid for every investment and change of investment he makes on your behalf. Guess why? You know the answer. The consultant who gets paid for every change is going to make a whole lot of changes whether or not they're good for you.

Here's my special tip on investments: keep it simple (plain vanilla stocks and bonds are the safest) and leave the other exotic stuff like options on futures and commodities to the Donald.

7. **Come to the love of your life with thoughts about financial solvency.** This is a big one. A woman who comes into marriage with a mind full of mush, saying, "Take care of my money, it's yours, I'm yours," is really a fool and inviting trouble. Dumbness about money is never cute and is a liability in the marriage, right off.

One of my biggest crusades now is teaching women how to manage their own money. Money management should be a requirement in school curriculums. The national debt is so high because too many kids stay kids throughout their adult life when it comes to finances.

It's imperative that you be grown-up about the money you make and hope to make; it's essential that you learn—before you tie the knot—how you wish to deal with finances. Come into marriage with ideas and beliefs. They can be wrong ideas, but at least they start dialogues and sharing about how finances should be handled. Such a dialogue can be whimsical and have little real substance, but it still gives couples a framework for how to begin. We don't have near enough money talk—money is almost taboo as a discussion topic, just as sex used to be. But if you dream together about a financial future, set goals, and make plans together, your chances of a loving marriage are so enhanced.

8. **Buy your home.** *The single most important thing any woman can do to prepare herself for financial soundness is to purchase her own home or apartment.*

Home ownership is almost the way America defines citizenship. If you own a home, you pay real estate taxes, and as long as you pay taxes, you have a vote within the municipality in which you live, a say in education in your area, a say in construction, a say in city hall, a say in the way you live your life. Financially, you build equity in yourself. Here are more advantages to home ownership:

- You build equity in property, and if you've bought in a good neighborhood, chances are excellent you'll always be able to sell at a profit. It's a way to build net worth as you make transitions from one home to the next.
- Home ownership allows you to go to banks and do many things like borrow to buy more property or send your kids to college or buy that boat.
- Very important is the fact that now you have tax breaks: you can deduct mortgage costs, interest and property taxes, and other expenditures on your tax return. If you've bought a rental property, you may be able to exclude capital gains taxes when you sell the property.

Here's the best thing: owning your home protects you against rent increases, which is a huge thing. You feel safe. Ownership gives you autonomy. No landlord can tell you, you can't hang this or install that. No one can tell you to be quiet. You can run naked through your house if you like, and no one can tell you to stop. It's empowering. Owning a home offers solace and protection to a woman alone.

One caveat: remember that even if a home is in your name alone, once you marry and live in the home with your husband, it belongs to both of you—not just you alone. It has become marital property, in many states and if you divorce, a portion of its worth belongs to your ex-husband as well as to you.

9. **Develop a financial record-keeping plan, and figure out a junk-throwing-away system.** This is *big*. I'm a compulsive neatnik, and it helps me enormously in money management. I keep almost everything because the more documentation you have, the more it serves as your credibility in any situation, whether it's contesting the IRS or applying for a bank loan. Still, you should be able to discard the now-worthless paper.

I have an excellent filing system. The best thing I can do for you is to say this: whenever you're in the grocery store, bookstore, or office supply store, go to the self-help section and for about five to fifteen bucks, pick up a book on budgeting that teaches you what to save and what to throw out, how to create folders, how to create labels, how to line things up in columns—not to mention how to budget your daily expenses. These magical little books help you define what you own, what you owe, what you need and don't need. They're organization plans, and these plans are invaluable when you're creating a financial road map to your future.

Just to give you an idea, here are some of the things you need to keep and file—sometimes forever:

- Records on home purchase and improvement
- Documents on stocks, bonds, jewelry, or art and any other assets you own
- Business expenses (for tax deductions—business meals, office expenses, bills paid, bills owed)

- Personal documents (birth certificates, marriage licenses, wills, deeds, titles, securities)
- Bank books, safe deposit records and keys, insurance policies, warranties for appliances, etc.

You need a filing system. Probably some sleek filing cabinets, also.

There are many books on the market, to help you organize this filing system. I happen to like *The Wall Street Journal Guide to Understanding Personal Finance*, which is sold in almost every bookstore.

10. **Ignore the thinking that says you're a threat to a guy if you have (and keep) your own money.** It's a myth and very wrong. Women become a threat to men only if they use their money in a controlling or demanding fashion. And we're not just talking about rich women—any woman, on any level, who manages her own finances wisely is a boon, not a threat to a smart man. If a guy is put off by your autonomy, he should be history in your life. It's good you found out how insecure such a man is before you got in too deeply.

11. **Retirement plans.** If you join a company 401 (k) or other retirement plan, contributing even $100 monthly can make you a millionaire before you know it. If your company matches your contributions, you'll be a double millionaire—because your company's investment in you is like getting a freebie every time you put in your own money. To save $200 before Uncle Sam taxes it is a gift your company gives you. At the end of the day you're only going to see a difference of about $20 from your paycheck. You're giving up $20 after taxes but receiving $200 before taxes. Figure it out.

You may be very far from retiring, but being ready for a commitment to another means you're also prepared to grow older together, comfortably; at sixty-two, it's no fun to have to scrape for movie money.

An Ordered Financial House—
If You Are Married or Planning Marriage

1. **Bottom line: Stay in control of what's yours, but share some, if you like.** Here is some of how Star and I did it.

   Everyone has shortcomings and weaknesses and, as a couple, Star and I decided to put out all our differences on the table and dig through that layer of vulnerability to see if we had a solid foundation underneath. We'd already decided we loved each other deeply; we stood solidly together in terms of our Christian beliefs. The big thing left was communication about how we spent and how we grew our money.

   For starters, I was younger than she, and she was in a more financially stable position. Was that going to have an effect on our relationship? You bet it was. For example, when I traveled, my budget said I stayed in a hotel room. *One* hotel room. But Star's budget and lifestyle said fancy suite of rooms. We had to discuss how we'd handle that situation so both of us would feel comfortable. Deciding, as anyone with a plan has to do, what was to be spent on normal household items went even further and extended to even the simplest things like, what products do you use in your house? I guarantee you, Star doesn't use plain old Dial soap. I do. If one uses much more expensive products than the other it can cause contention in a relationship. Deal with it. Lay out your differences, and plan how you're going to deal with all possible expenditures.

2. **The Prenup.** I think every woman, especially a woman with financial resources of her own, should expect to create a prenuptial agreement with her prospective husband. Certainly, Star and I made a prenup: I insisted upon it.

   The prenup says, in case of death or divorce, whatever you bring to the table is yours and will always be yours. Whatever you owned, whatever you inherited, whatever you saved in your name alone before the marriage can stay yours alone. If you are widowed or divorced and have a substantial estate, it's crucial to have a prenup, not least because you want to preserve your own money for your children of previous marriages. If one partner comes into the marriage with much more financial buildup than the other, he or she should want a prenup for obvious reasons. Remember, though, *a home you may own yourself and then live in together after the marriage becomes marital property* (and not yours alone anymore).

That's the kit and caboodle—unless you both specify in your prenup that you want something different. And also remember that the prenup agreement covers only money issues, not who vacuums the rug or walks the dog. Each of you, by the way, must have your own lawyer in drawing up a prenup. Be scrupulously honest in declaring what each owns before you sign any agreement: not being straight about finances can make the prenup null and void should one of you decide to contest it.

3. **Straight-talk time.** Now, before the wedding, discuss what each of you earns, owns, and owes. Discuss what could happen after a baby is born or if one person loses a job. Discuss if you'll invest together or if each will invest on her or his own. Talk about health and life insurance and what you need. Talk about what financial responsibilities each of you has: does either of you owe money to an institution or a family member—where will it come from? Does one or both of you have ailing parents who require financial help? Does one of you plan to go back to school—and how will that be paid for? Lay it all out on that table.

4. **Brokerage accounts.** If a woman has created her own accounts from her own money (or money her family has given her as gifts), I believe it should remain her own. Later, if she marries and wishes to add her husband to the account in some way, that can be negotiated, but she still remains in control of the bulk of her assets.

5. **Your own accounts.** Let's start with checking accounts, regular interest-bearing checking accounts. Every woman definitely needs a checking account in her own name, as does every man. We're talking grown-ups here—no one should have to go to anyone else to ask for money for private and personal expenditures or for simple mad

money. Each fills the private accounts with his or her own earned money. If one partner is a stay-at-home parent and doesn't earn money, it doesn't mean she or he should have no private account. The one who is earning the cash for the family puts an equal amount in each of the private checking accounts (it's only fair), and that amount should be decided upon together.

6. **A shared account.** If you are married or in a committed relationship, you should also share a checking account for the household. The joint household account is filled by a percentage of each person's earnings: when earnings are unequal (if he makes $100,000 and she makes $20,000), he donates five times as much as she. Joint checking accounts, by the way, have an added virtue in that each spouse's spending habits are pretty much out in the open—a good thing.

7. **Who pays what?** Next, both of you decide in advance who pays the bills. Decide how you're going to divide expenses. Some people decide that all personal purchases should come out of your own account and all household expenses come out of the shared account. Others think differently. The important thing is to discuss it all and agree.

   If the bill is a household bill, you've also decided in advance who actually picks up the pen to pay what from the joint account (it's a good idea to let just one of you handle the mutual bills). This creates structure in a relationship and, in my mind, is a defined plan. We want to avoid questions like, Why didn't you pay the phone bill? Why are the credit cards maxed out? Why have we gotten a second notice on the electric bill?

8. **Mention to the other that you're buying a boat. Or a mink coat.** It's a big mistake not to share your major financial decisions with each other—even if the money comes from your personal account. If I bought a boat without telling Star, let me tell you that boat would probably go straight back. Not that she works the same way, to be frank. Once, she came home with a fur coat.

   "Where did that thing come from, baby?" I asked.

   "Oh, it's just a little something I found on the way home," she answered.

"Okay, sweetheart," I sighed.

Although every guy is not such a doll as I, I can still promise you that nine times out of ten, if you just communicate, talk about the big item purchase before you make it, the other will most likely agree.

9. **Does the person who makes more money get to call the shots?** Honestly? Most of the time, yes. It's how people are taught, and it's one of the toughest things to deal with in any relationship. But, it doesn't have to be that way. Depending on how easily you communicate with your partner, you can together decide if the good stuff the other brings to the marriage (taking care of the kids, managing the home and arranging the social life, getting educated so you can be a full financial equal) should count as points in any financial decision-making process facing you as a couple. Star and I have a plan that factors out the control issue. If there's a need in the house, we have to both agree that it has to be taken care of. Then, we both agree on what portion each pays, according to his or her capacity. We treat our financial issues almost like a corporation, and that seems to factor out who's made more money that year.

10. **Red-flag guys.** I thought a couple of words would be in order here on red-flag behavior in men—guys you should avoid because they almost definitely do not have their own financial houses in order. Avoid a guy . . .
    - who never has any money in his pocket, who can't even tip the garage guy. Run as fast as possible.
    - who doesn't have a credit card. Run.
    - who answers his own phone and often says, "He doesn't live here anymore." You know those are creditors calling. Run.
    - who never even answers his home phone and tells you not to pick up, either. Run.
    - who seems to get an inordinate amount of mail from credit card companies. Run.

11. **The passing down.** You meet someone, you fall in love, you make a commitment to marry, you marry. You are going to be together a long, long time—you hope and pray. You've talked about what you hope to

accomplish in the next two to three years, the next three to seven years, the next ten plus years. It makes great financial sense also to talk about what you hope will be your legacy to children, family, or friends. A discussion about transferring wealth is a way of making your bond even stronger.

A great way to find out about how to best transfer wealth is to attend your local high school, college, library, or church group seminars on the subject. They're free and they're informative and can give you tools (making a will is the easiest one) that will help you connect to future generations. You'll need a trusts and estates attorney to make your wishes legal.

*   *   *

This is me, Star, talking now: thank you, Al.

It filled me with a great sense of security to know that my man cared passionately about our family finances and the financial future of our family.

Approaching the money discussion can be a scary prospect, but *not* discussing it prior to marriage will lead to doing *nothing but* discussing it during marriage. Our plan is in place, all we have to do now is follow it . . . and I have to remember to check with my husband the next time I want a new fur coat.

Chapter 7

Sex and Dating in a Moral Context

Be humble for you are made of earth.
Be noble for you are made of stars.

SERBIAN PROVERB

S o, this is how I met a man made of earth and stars—when I was finally ready.

We had a contest on *The View,* and one of the viewers won the "Star Treatment," which was to get treated like a star while spending the day with me. She got her first-ever massage, facial, manicure, and pedicure, and I took her to her first red carpet event—a fabulous party to celebrate the launch of Alicia Keys's new album. On November 13, 2003, at a New York studio, during the glitzy launch with my guest, Stephanie Guillen, from Denver, Colorado, right by my side, I saw my friend Anthony (my lawyer's husband) across the room and went over to hug him hello. After a few words, distracted, I started to leave when a man standing near Anthony reached out, took my arm, and said, "You're not just going to pass me by."

I looked up—and was floored. This handsome man with skin the color of cooked butter, this man with the most beautiful lips I'd ever seen, a Clark Gable jawline, and the deepest brown eyes on the planet softly continued what he'd started to say, which was, "I saw you once at a party five years ago and was too hesitant to approach you, but this time, I'm braver."

I was charmed out of my wits. I stopped, looked into those chocolate eyes, and I literally heard a bell ring—just like my mother said it would. This time it was a bell of exultation, not warning. Not to be corny . . . but I *exhaled.*

When I walked into that room the day I met Al Scales Reynolds, I didn't walk in with the intention of meeting someone. I walked in with my mind on feeling good about me. I was prepared. I'd started on getting ready. My relationship with God was strong, my health was getting better by the day, and my weight-loss program had been moving along for months. When that tall, smart, wonderful man took my arm, I was emotionally, physically, and spiritually ready to accept him. I deserved him. And you know what? I wasn't looking for him—*he* was looking for me.

Not Looking for Temporary

From then on, everything about our relationship has been steeped in romance. On date one, Al presented me with a CD of songs each with the word *star* in them.

But more important was date two.

Picture it.

We'd gone to church together at eight in the morning and had come back to my apartment for a home-cooked meal. Al was sitting on the floor in my living room, having changed into his fraternity sweatpants, the *New York Times* was strewn all over, and football was blaring on the television. I came out of my room, having changed into my own sweats, stood in the doorway looking at the scene, and saw my life as I'd always dreamed it would be.

"This is what it feels like to be ready," I thought. "Sunday after church, something good-smelling in the kitchen, football on TV, and Al lounging on the floor." I felt myself grinning at him from the doorway.

He smiled back, stood up, took my hands, and said the words I'll never forget as long as I may live.

"I'm not looking for temporary," he said. "And I don't want short-term. What are you trying to do?"

"What do you mean?" I asked. I was trembling.

"I mean," he said, "I'm no longer interested in playing around. I want *her* in my life, and if you're not *her,* we can be friends, but I'm no longer interested in silly relationships that lead nowhere."

I thought I'd heard myself coming back on myself. Whooooaaaa.

"Well, you have to know I'm also not interested in sport dating," I answered. From that moment on, we started thinking of ourselves as two parts of a penny— heads and tails—total simpatico. My girlfriend Vanessa said to me, "I know why you moved forward with Al so quickly; it was because you'd been in the game long enough to know what isn't right."

She was right-on. When what was good came along and I was ready, it was so obvious—it was like night and day compared to the other relationships I'd had.

And—that romance. We'd talk on the phone till four o'clock in the morning. He asked about my hopes and dreams, and I'd ask about his plans for the future. He said I love you for the first time when he sent flowers to *The View* for me.

I sent flowers to his Wall Street office. He sent me daily love notes by fax. I left singing messages on his voice mail. He covered the floor of my living room with a trail of roses. You want to know why I was giddy with love? It was all his fault.

Within a month of our meeting, we headed to each other's hometowns, where we met with both families. We needed to see each other's roots, observe each other's witnesses. In December, we seriously began discussing marriage and commitment. We told our families about our feelings, and we told my pastor, A. R. Bernard from the Christian Cultural Center in Brooklyn, New York. He began talking to us about love and commitment and fidelity. For the first time in my life, I wasn't frightened about what was happening.

And it was happening fast. We planned to spend Valentine's Day at the NBA All-Star Game in Los Angeles. Al picked me up at the TV studio, and we headed, I thought, to the airport, but no—it appeared the car was heading back toward my house. He'd forgotten something he needed. The whole way home, I was "flapping those jaws," as Al likes to say.

Coming into my apartment, I stopped short. The dining room was set with champagne, hors d'oeuvres, and flowers. I continued talking and fussing as I walked into the living room, and there they were, my whole family—parents, sister, and nephews. Al had brought them all to New York so they could be present at this vital moment in my life. I couldn't believe it.

He dropped to one knee and promised to love me the rest of my life.

You gotta love a guy like that.

Then, he gave me a promise ring.

What? That didn't thrill me. The engagement ring was going to come in LA, he said, when he "formally" asked me to marry him. I wanted to know when. He told me I'd have to wait and see.

At the Staples Center in Los Angeles, the buzzer rang out, starting the fourth quarter of the game, and Al again dropped to one knee in front of TV viewers and twenty thousand screaming fans and asked me to be his wife.

I said yes. Actually, I said it six times—"Yesyesyesyesyesyes!"

By the way—you know that day I told you about when Al arranged to have my family in New York when he asked for my hand in marriage? I found out later (from my mother, not from Al) that Al took my parents to breakfast that morning and laid out our future for them. He told them about his finances, his hopes, his dreams, and his plans for us as a couple. He had of course discussed these subjects with me, but to know that he had the strength of character to have the discussion with my parents prior to asking me to be his wife filled me with a wonderful sense of security and love. He's the real thing—I know it like I know my name.

How Do You Really Know if He's the One?

I used to date a guy who was wonderful, but he despised sports. He could not sit down and watch a basketball game with me for anything. I could never have married him any more than I could have married a guy with no spirituality in his heart. After Al and I were married, there came one Sunday afternoon during the NBA finals. Al had been traveling; I was coming back from the Hamptons. We met at the door, undressed, and got into our bed and turned on the Pistons and the Spurs and sat there and yelled at the TV. "Baby, what is wrong with him?

What is that kind of shot?" That was Al. And I'm going back at him, "Oh, please, they're not playing team ball. That's the problem!" And we're going back and forth, back and forth, and back and forth. I could not have lived without that back and forth.

Bishop T. D. Jakes of the Potter's House, a nondenominational church in Dallas, Texas, once gave a sermon in which he was trying to explain to a group of young women how you could pick and choose the man in your life. "How do you know that he's *the one?*" asked Bishop Jakes.

And then, that great spiritual leader answered his own question.

"I'll tell you how you know if he's the one. I want you to close your eyes and think of the very worst day of your life, the day you lower one of your parents into the ground. Doesn't get any worse than that, does it? Doesn't get any worse. Your mama, the person who's always there for you, put into the ground. Now, the guy you're seeing? Is he the guy who's standing there next to you with his arm around you? If you can't see him there on that bad day, he ain't the one."

I can honestly tell you from the moment I met Al, I knew that on that bad day when I could not hold myself up, he'd be the one who would hold me up. I could not imagine another person holding me up.

Here are four other ways you can tell if he's the one:

1. **Does he keep you company?** My guy does. This is the silly answer of how I knew he'd keep me company. We'd been dating only two weeks, and I was getting my hair braided in my bedroom by three West African women. They'd brushed all my hair out, and it was in that half-and-half stage—half-braided, half looking crazy, you know—long, flowing, wild. I sighed with impatience because if truth be told, my feet hurt. Al was watching a ball game in the living room, but all of a sudden, there he was in my room. And he started massaging my feet while Fifi and the girls braided my hair. The entire time I was getting my hair braided, he lay across the bed, and we laughed, and we watched TV, and he kept me company—and it was a sign of things to come, Al keeping me company when I have a headache, when I'm sad, when I'm tense, and certainly when I'm happy. Don't worry. I do the same for him.

2. **Does he gentle his criticisms?** Sometimes, Al has to stand firm when

I'm in my very bossy mode, but he rarely criticizes me without starting with the words "sweetheart" or "babe." As in, "Babe, think about it this way." Or, "Sweetheart, I think there might be another option here." His sweetness just mellows me out.

3. **Does he push your hot buttons?** I'm not talking about the ones that make you *hot,* I'm talking about the ones that make you mad and always hurt the most. During premarital counseling, we learned about each other's hot buttons. Al knows the location of each of my buttons, and he chooses not to go there. That's a big deal. We have no excuses about being accidentally mean to each other because we can't say, "I didn't know that would piss you off." We do know; we know everything about the other. Sometimes, thinking like a lawyer can have its negative side. I am very good at wrangling. My mother once told me I don't fight fairly because when I'm angry I'll tend to push the button that will most injure you. But when you love someone, you don't want to jab deeply because it hurts you to see his pain. I can almost literally see Al's heart when he's angry and is tempted to say something to dig me (hey, girl, it happens!), but he always chooses not to go there. That really makes him the one.

4. **Does he love and respect his mom or the women in his life?** You may disagree with me on this one, but a man who treats other women kindly, especially his mother, is usually a nice person. That's important.

Personal Stuff

The things I'm about to tell you next are really quite intimate and personal, but I've decided to do it because they go to the heart of my heart. Ordinarily, I'm pretty close mouthed about my private life, but I want to be totally candid here. I also want to say that although I'm convinced that the way we came to deal with sexuality and morality before our marriage is the most wonderful way, still, it is our way and it may not be yours. That's fine—we each find our own path. But, oh, how it's worked for us.

Most of my girlfriends are Christian, and even those who aren't have a certain spirituality that sustains them through everything. We often talked about the dynamic of dating as adult women and having physical and emotional needs met during this time, but still wanting—and usually failing—to be obedient to God's word to have sex only within the context of marriage. Back and forth, and back and forth we've debated this point. It is true that at many given times, some of us had taken on short periods of celibacy. Maybe we were between boyfriends. Maybe we felt we'd just gotten out of a crappy relationship and needed to take a break. Then, there are some women who just can't be without a man—I don't know if it's physical or emotional. There are a whole lot of reasons.

One of our best reasons, we thought, for *not* being celibate was that most of us were not kids, and we'd arrived at that stage in life where sexuality seemed too easy and too natural to ration it out.

We were wrong. If you really think about it, there should be defined stages to any relationship that's going to last beyond the "running toward each other in slow motion" phase. The "wham, bam, let's fall into bed" mentality was easy, but it wasn't working for most of us. Our relationships were shallow, and the sex wasn't all that great. One night in Bible study, Pastor Bernard shared a heavy concept with the bible study group that Al and I attended, and a lightbulb went off in my head. Sexual intimacy ought to be earned, we learned; a relationship is better primed to last when friends, not strangers, fall into bed.

The stages Pastor Bernard talked about are described below: when you skip any one stage to jump ahead in the relationship, I think you're setting yourself up for failure.

Stages of a Lasting Relationship

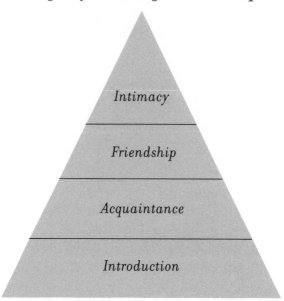

I can't tell you how long each stage should last—God knows I was on warp speed with Al—but I do know that each stage is separate and distinct and provides a snapshot of the relationship's future. This is the way Al and I figured it should be broken down.

The introduction stage: This is the getting-to-know-each-other part. Where are you from, what is your background, who raised you, how were you raised, what's your profession—all this comes out in the introductory stage.

The acquaintance stage: Now you find out what you have in common. Do you both like sports (is it basketball, tennis, or football—be specific!), or do you both adore theater? Do you share a faith—is it important to you—or not? Do you both like to talk for hours on the phone, or do you avoid the phone like the plague? This vital stage allows you to disclose your habits, likes, dislikes, and strong beliefs with the other. Do you mesh, do you match? This is the time when you discover if you really enjoy the other enough to spend a whole lot of time with him.

The friendship stage: Hitting this phase of the relationship means you're really starting to cook with gas. This is the time you find out if you can depend on each other; do you have each other's backs? How do you feel about loyalty and friendships and family? Can you share emotionally? Do you have a similar life plan? Do you reallyreallyreallyreallyreally like/love the other? This was my favorite stage with Al, during which he became my best friend and confidant. That's why, when we finally became intimate, the sexuality was born of hopes, dreams, and love in addition to desire.

Finally, the intimacy stage: Joining your bodies along with your hearts. If you've completed each stage, you have no doubt of who the *person* is inside the body you're joining. Your heart, mind, and soul are already one with his. Once I really understood that, I couldn't argue with the whole concept of stages.

I couldn't stop thinking of a sermon I once heard years and years ago that stuck with me. Every time a woman shares her body with a man, the pastor had said, the man literally leaves part of himself. If you share your body in an irresponsible way, there will come a time when you are filled with others—and there's no room for you. There's no room for you.

I always thought about that. I didn't want to get to that point where I no longer had room for me.

Flash backward: I should tell you that when I started preparing myself for meeting the man God wanted me to have, I'd independently decided to cleanse myself emotionally and physically of every other man. First, I'd stopped comparing every man I met to other men. I never talked about whether another guy was good or wasn't good to me (as in "my ex-boyfriend used to . . ."). No new relationship, I decided, needed to have the baggage of an old relationship weighing it down.

Then, I wanted also to cleanse myself physically of every other man. Although I didn't yet know the man of my dreams was close, I still, all by myself, had determined to start a period of celibacy—temporary abstinence. I was in the process of losing a significant amount of weight, and I wasn't even in the mood for sex. I was trying to take care of me, physically. The thought had come to me: maybe, just maybe the next person I get involved with was going to be the one. I wanted to be clean and new for him.

Soon after, there he was—Al. I have to be honest: at once, I felt tremendously passionate, wildly attracted to him. We didn't sleep together the first night, but he stayed all night, and we talked about that scene from *Waiting to Exhale* where Wesley Snipes and Angela Bassett ended up sleeping on top of the covers in their clothes. It was a very romantic and sexy—though celibate—scene. I wondered out loud, that first night with Al, if there would ever be a guy I'd feel so connected to in that way. He didn't answer.

After our date in church that Sunday, he and I each went away to be with our families for Thanksgiving. And then, we came home.

Wow. I can hardly think of that next week without shaking. Out the window went my temporary abstinence. I was wildly, madly, passionately in love.

We went out dirty dancing—we call it slow dragging—four nights in a row. That's when the music makes your body gyrate, and you just want to be in each other's arms. It was all so intense and lusty, and the first time ever he held me in his arms sexually, it was so urgent and almost frightening for both of us because we knew our erotic interest in each other could take over every other single thing.

So, we had an intimate, intoxicatingly sexual connection the first two months of our relationship. We traveled to Jamaica together, and I had someone who wanted to be there just for me. With Al, I walked on the beach for the first time in my adult life without getting winded. We walked a mile, and we talked and talked seriously about marriage, just by ourselves and then, even with other people. We talked about what it meant—that commitment—and we made the decision that because we knew this was all moving too quickly, we wanted to bring a spiritual adviser into the relationship.

It wasn't an easy decision. We both knew the first thing he'd say was, "To test this relationship and be obedient, you must be celibate until marriage."

But before we walked into that meeting with Pastor Bernard, we ourselves decided that Jamaica would be the last time we were sexually intimate with each other until the night of our wedding.

So the pastor said . . .

"The first thing you have to do to test this relationship," said Pastor Bernard, "is to be obedient and celibate until marriage." He told us that this period before our marriage should be a time of abstinence and fidelity for us because it would, in many ways, insure our ability to be faithful after marriage.

"Things are going to come up," said our pastor, "that are going to test your ability for fidelity. If you can't be faithful to a six-month vow of abstinence, what are you going to do if something really intense happens in your marriage? This is a time to find out if you want him, not just his body, if you want her, not just her body."

His words reverberated with us. We knew what they meant. We knew we had to be ready. If you just want a lover, you don't have to be so ready, but if you want a husband and not just a lover—and I did—you have to begin the relationship the way you want it to be forever. I wanted a man who would respect my being obedient to my own values. I wanted a man who would be strong in character and faith. I wanted someone who would look at me and feel immense attraction but have the strength of character to contain it at the appropriate time. God forbid I should be disabled or have a toxic pregnancy or for some other reason not be able to have sex. Would my husband still want me, would he be able to stay faithful during trying times?

We talked for hours and hours, and vowed that we did want to be faithful throughout our marriage in mind, body, and spirit. We kind of looked at it as a challenge. We would see if we could break boundaries and old patterns of behavior and not use sexuality as the only means of connection. In my old life, when it was too hard to talk, too hard to explain, too hard to fight, sometimes I'd used my body as a means to communicate. I wanted to find other ways beyond sex to communicate. We both wanted to build up the tenderness that is sometimes lost in the actual sex act.

We took the vow.

Here's the fascinating part. Right after our pastor offered us that call to arms, we started getting intensely personal, mean-spirited media attention—attacks on our character, on our sexuality, on everything—nasty, vicious attacks clearly designed to hurt our relationship. Why? I have no idea. Maybe it was because I was truly obnoxious as I publicly talked about how happy I was during this time. I was in the throes of a love that I'd never before experienced. I was becoming physically fit for the first time. My spirit was soaring with a new dedication to Christ. Life was good.

For some, it must have sounded too good, even like bragging, because, in all honesty, people we didn't even know spent months of their lives trying to ruin ours. I don't really know why certain people are so mean. All I know is that their terrible wrath was hurting our hearts.

There's an old Chinese proverb that does not speak to my Christian values but still gave me some comfort during those times: "I sit by the bank of the river and wait for the body of my enemy to float by." I knew that if I just waited, all these mean people, these radio shock jocks and mean-spirited gossip mavens would get theirs—they always do. Still, the attacks were so relentless. I had trouble just sitting by the bank of the river waiting; I'm an action person. But I had Al—and I had our growing connection.

I swear an oath that I couldn't have gotten through that terrible period of time had Al and I not had learned the many other ways of comforting each other that we had to learn when we took a vow to be temporarily abstinent. We would not be married today.

Desire doesn't go away when you take a vow of temporary abstinence. That's why, in order for it to work, you absolutely need other outlets to satisfy your sexual appetite. Al and I often used dancing as that outlet. We would play our favorite albums—*Kemistry* or *The Diary of Alicia Keys*—or we would listen to the soul singer Anthony Hamilton. We'd find songs and give them as gifts to each other, and listen as we held hands. We'd read poetry out loud. When I say to you that this was far more intense lovemaking than any "wham, bam, thank you ma'am" could ever be, I mean it. We'd learned that we could talk and those talks would be comforting. We learned how to whisper silliness in each other's ears, go out to dinner with our heads held high, write each other poems, spend hours in a card shop to find the exact right card that would get the other through the emotional meanness to which we were being subjected. We couldn't rely on sex because we'd taken that vow. So, we learned how to have everything else. You know what we did? We learned how to make love without having sexual intercourse. It would hold us for a while.

And we were so very intimate within the bonds of our vow. Because we were in love and very sexual and had already experienced intercourse, we wanted to keep that level of intimacy without breaking our vow. We learned things that some couples married thirty years don't know—how to dedicate ourselves to each other so nothing in the outside world could ever pierce that. No one could get into our smallest, inner circle.

Our close friends, staff, and colleagues protected us—they were that second circle of people who also knew of our vow of obedience. But every single day, television programs still had something nasty to say; we were in the gossip columns of newspapers and magazines every single week. The Internet was particularly brutal.

We once did a segment on *The View* with teenagers who had been harassed on the Internet. Their classmates had spent months tormenting them with such vicious, made-up, horribly untrue gossip on the Net, they needed professional help to get through it. After the segment, I spoke privately with the teens and told them I knew what they were feeling because I'd also experienced that same kind of relentless name-calling. I wanted them to know that if this forty-something woman felt her spirit crushed by such bullying, these kids had to be devastated.

By the way, bullying often doesn't stop when you graduate from high school. Sometimes the bullies follow you right into your adult life, and their purpose remains identical to their eleventh-grade agenda: they want you to feel as bad about yourself as they feel about themselves, and so they try to rob you of your joy in life. I told these young teens not to falter: their greatest revenge would be to live well and be happy.

Absolute
〜
What doesn't kill you makes you stronger.

I have to admit it: I was having trouble handling the viciousness. I guess my armor was pierced deeper than I wanted anyone to know, but Al knew, and in the midst of it all, he put his foot down and said, "We will *not* have any negative coming into our home; no one may bring mean magazines or newspapers into this cherished place."

I told the teens the story of how we dealt with it, and I'll tell you.

If there was something mean or nasty that we had to deal with publicly (and there was a lot of it), we'd go to a restaurant, discuss it, decide on a game plan, execute the plan, and then close it off from the rest of our lives. It was the only way we remained sane.

Again—I have to say it twice—I would not be married today had I not made up my mind that my physical and emotional connection to Al was so much more long term than those six months in which we were to be sexually celibate together.

Temporary abstinence can be kind of a quiet, resting state, a temporary fast that forces you to find other emotional outlets. Eventually, it makes you even hungrier for sexual intercourse, but hungrier for a full meal, not fast food.

The first two months we were celibate, it was kind of whimsical for us—like, "Ooooh—look at this, we're doin' it." I mean, Al is a beautiful man. He's got the legs of a stallion. He'd be a perfect Ralph Lauren model—you take something off the rack, put it on that body, and it's going to look dreamy. When you're a young brown-skinned girl growing up in the South, you dream of marrying the light-skinned black boy with the curly hair, and he's Prince Charming from when you were like seven years old. And I'd chosen to be celibate with this man! Whoaaaa.

But we both probably had the hardest time during the next two months because we were traveling a lot and it became very intense, and we were far from home and family. There were days we were both emotionally drained—no, I was more like depressed and sad, but intense prayer and our ability to communicate on other levels than just through intercourse moved us through this period. Still, we were convinced more than ever that we wanted a four-course gourmet dinner, not a McDonald's burger, so we stuck with it. The last two months of our temporary fast, we grew even closer together than I'd ever dreamed possible. We set a template for talking about almost everything—which is essential in any marriage. We had the time to do it.

There's wonderment in Al that I love—as if a new thing has just happened when he sees an old thing that strikes him as wonderful. Al knows museums and great art and architecture and finance. He's not so good at pop culture. There are great movies he's never seen or even heard of. But I know pop culture, and I drew him into that world in which there are things that are maybe not so great, but, honey, great to me—stuff I wanted to teach him about. Like, my favorite TV show is *Law and Order*. I watch every one. At that, he rebelled. My husband heard *dum dum,* and he'd say, "I can't be in this room with you because then I've got to hear that *dum dum* again, and it means *Law and Order* is coming on."

But sometimes, secretly, he found himself getting caught up in the story. Then within five minutes, he'd say, "Baby—I'm just confused, why would they do that?"

And I'd have to explain to him, it's just television's dramatic license. In the end, we learned to share all this and have such fun doing it because we were taking a vacation from sex. I'm convinced of it.

Actually, the final weeks of our vow were a piece of cake because we saw the home stretch and were planning the wedding.

The Wedding

I wish I had the power to describe to other women the feeling I had when I was getting ready on my wedding day, making all the intimate preparations that women who have traditionally done through the ages as they get ready for intimacy. I had taken a long bath, had a sensuous massage and a gorgeous body scrub. I put on lingerie that my husband-to-be had never seen, and applied scented oil and creams he'd never smelled on my body. As I prepared, I can remember listening to music and smiling, and I felt a bond with brides of centuries ago.

And finally, I'm at the back of the church in my long, white dress, and I see Al looking at me way at the end of the aisle, and *his face was magnificent.* The only thing I could think of is that if anything ever goes wrong, I'll always have this moment. I saw his face and I knew we'd done what we'd said we were going to do, and I was filled with love.

Give me chastity . . . but not just now.

ST. AUGUSTINE

If you think you want to try a temporary celibacy, unlike St. Augustine, now, today is the time to start. Let me help you. Here's what it takes to do it:

Remember—it's never too late

Biblically, you're supposed to come to your husband having not known anyone else. Yeahhhhh, right. Once you reach a certain adult age—I was forty—that nice thought may be just a fleeting memory and impossible. But you can decide at any age to cleanse yourself of past relationships, to be pure for true love to come.

Only date guys who respect your views: look for them in all the right places

The last thing you want to do is have a fight with the new man in your life every time he feels amorous. I've said it a million times, and here it is again: you've got to find a guy who shares your core values, and I'm not just talking about sexuality. You've got to move in tandem with the man of your dreams, share deep beliefs. Even if you come from a blue state and he from a red state, you've got to find ease, not friction, in talking about your differences. Make no mistake: there *will* be differences—no man is your clone. But differences in opinion ought to make life together more intoxicating, not more stress filled.

Go looking for such a man in places where you want to end up together. For example, if you love sports as I do, then you should hang out at sporting events where like-minded men will be found, and where you wish to be found after you meet the guy of your dreams. If you like volunteerism, join a board in a local community organization because you'll meet men and women there who think as you do. Participate in annual charity events, luncheons, and dinners, and volunteer to serve on a committee. Volunteer to do something you've never done before—organize a fund-raiser, edit a newsletter for a neighborhood group. Step outside your box and look around for others who have done the same thing.

For example, I'm very involved with the Rush Philanthropic Arts Foundation Art for Life projects founded by our friends Russell and Kimora Lee Simmons. Art for Life brings the visual and performing arts into the lives of children from low-income communities. Although this is good enough reason for you to get involved in the amazing organization, you can't imagine how many attractive single men also belong. I also participate in Girls Incorporated because I'm interested in mentoring young women, and you might also volunteer in such a group or your local Boys and Girls Club because there are many swell men who also volunteer. Volunteer to help staff a political base of your choosing during election fever: I guarantee you there will be nice men looking for *you* at these venues. Try something new—take a writing or a photography course, take a nature walk. Attend services at your local church, synagogue, or mosque if you feel spiritual pulls to these groups—and assume there will be single guys present feeling the same pull.

I do not think you should go at all of this with the sole goal of meeting a man. That puts too much pressure of the wrong sort upon your shoulders, and trying new things is a huge reward all by itself. But if you enlarge your life and enhance your heart and soul with participation in such activities, a like-minded guy with whom you can be equally yoked sitting right near you would be a strong possibility (more on yoking on page 149).

If he's the right guy, he will go with you on the same journey. If he's not the right guy, it's better you find out now.

Don't advertise what's not on the market

I believe when a woman says no, it's no, but it's still your responsibility not to send mixed signals. If you want to remain celibate, don't wear the low-cut blouses and tight pants that may be misinterpreted. And need I say it, keep your clothes on. Be responsible for the messages you convey. Now, with my husband, I wear some of the tightest jeans on the planet and very low cut T-shirts, and I'm aware that sometimes when he's talking to me, he's talking right to my chest. But when you're ready for true love, if you feel you want to enter into a temporary abstinence from sex to purify yourself, refresh your sexual desire, or learn to experience the joys of love in alternate ways—you can wait to wear the sexy clothes and speak in sex-laden doublespeak. You can wait for the tight jeans, even wait for the Manolo Blahnik high heels. Their time will come.

Keep control—of drugs, alcohol, and mouth

Before I met Al, I had one big rule that I followed without exception: never go out drinking in a public place without somebody along with you. I liked to refer to that person as my wingman, someone who's on my wing, who has my back. That way, if your wingman (who also can be your best girlfriend) sees you're drinking a little too much, or notices that someone else has slipped a little inducement into your drink, or you're starting to sound a little louder or more sexy than usual, she's going to say, "Okay, Kendra, let's go." And, if you don't have a girlfriend, get one. Sitting at a bar by yourself puts you in a vulnerable, potentially out-of-control situation.

And remember, I'm a big old prude, the last forty-three-year-old in America who's never smoked a joint, but if you do, have Kendra there to watch your back so you don't end up looking like Party Girl Central, when all you want to do is have fun. If you're acting like those girls on *Girls Gone Wild* videotapes and flashing your breasts to the camera, and a man comes over and touches you inappropriately, well, you need to expect that you've told him you're a Girl Gone Wild. Okay?

And the mouth: don't use foul language—certainly when in new relationships. Don't throw out come-on, cutesy phrases. It says stuff about you that may or may not be true, but can't be helpful in retaining your celibacy.

If you have a failure experience, if you slip and do the deed and hate yourself in the morning . . .

Start all over. The Bible says that a just man can fail seven times—I translate that into a just woman can also fail seven times. If you go back with a penitent heart, you can start all over. But you can't go back and say, "Okay, I slipped on Tuesday, and I'm going to slip again on Thursday because this really cute guy asked me out . . ." No, noooo, darling, that's not a penitent heart.

Remember the benefits—especially when you're tempted

Number one benefit: You can prove to yourself that you're in control of your body—a nice thing for any woman to know.

Number two benefit: Temporary abstinence opens doors to new ways of love and lovemaking. It actually enhances the physical act of sexual intercourse—*when* you're ready.

Number three benefit: You can stop worrying about AIDS, venereal disease, or pregnancy.

Okay—there are other ways

One last word about all this: it'll come as no shock to realize you can certainly enjoy dating in a moral context, even if you don't subscribe to my temporary abstinence view. Still, when you're preparing to meet a man with whom you can fruitfully spend the rest of your life, *know that it still helps to be as good a girl as you can manage.* You know what a good girl is, you know when you are acting the way you hope your daughter would act. I don't have to spell that out, children, do I?

What I can say without reservation is that *everyone* should subscribe to certain basic tenets of making great, lasting moral connections.

An unlikely person recently said it best:

The CEO Speaks

Here's some relationship advice I love even though it comes from an unusual source, Jack Welch, the legendary chairman and chief executive officer of General Electric, who has had his own share of glare in this area. He says that intimate relationships should be managed in the same way great business relationships are managed, and that is with candor, transparency, and celebration. This is what I think he means.

Candor

Be straight, be honest with the men you date, and you have the best chance of ending up in a morally responsible relationship. I believe that you must never be afraid to say what's in your heart and mind—even if it's not particularly flattering to a date or politically correct. Sometimes, I guess, I get in trouble with that in my public life, but truth telling has always been a great road to travel with the men in my life. Heck, if I did it even more, I probably wouldn't have screwed up so much. I like people whom I *might* eventually love to know how I feel about things. What's the point of wasting time acting like someone you're not?

There's one caveat here: if you give out your truths, you must also be prepared for the other person to come right back at you with his honesty. Take it on, sister—listen to the brother. It's like being a sponge and that's cool: as a sponge, you can soak up all the stuff you need, and then, wring out the excess. You can wring and wring and wring, but you'll never wring a sponge dry—you'll always retain enough to clean those windows! Give your truths, accept his, retain what is good—then stay if you wish, move on, if you wish. In whatever direction you go, candor will see you home.

Transparency

Don't be afraid to allow a good man to see your vulnerable side. Don't be afraid to give up the reins every once in a while. This was pretty hard for me to learn. In my controlling way, I didn't want to make myself too vulnerable, too transparent because I thought I needed a nine-foot-high wall to protect me from being hurt. Then, I finally realized that if I did the thing I believe one should do in a relationship—make sure you're with someone who shares your values—then that person's not going to grab your gift of transparency and run away with your secrets, he's not going to hurt you. Here's a little-known fact: you tell a secret about yourself, you probably get one back from him, about him. Transparency leads to solidity in a relationship.

Here's a secret about me that I had a hard time sharing with Al, a secret that many women will criticize me for—I just know it. But here goes:

I'm a Southern girl. I was raised to believe that if you marry a man worthy of you, you accept him as your *priest* (the person who leads your family and worship), your *prophet* (he's the one who knows best where we're going as a family), and your *king* (he takes the lead). So, get this picture: I'm this big powerful prosecuting attorney, this mouthy television star, and I feel—if you're a man that's worthy of me, will you take the lead?

I may be many things but I'm not dumb, and I know this attitude is not popular with my fellow feminists and with many men, as well. It actually puts a great burden on men—being the one who has to make most of the decisions in the family. Many men have gotten used to women taking that burden from them.

You know what? The thing that has probably shocked me the most in public reactions to my marriage has been the snarky comments—especially from women—about my taking Al's last name, as in Star Jones *Reynolds*. Despite the fact that a 2004 Harvard University study indicates that since the year 2000 most young women with university degrees are alarming older feminists by indeed taking their husband's last names (even though before that, the clear trend was to retain their maiden names), I keep hearing, "What's with this Star Jones *Reynolds?*"

But I love living with his name.

Although I choose that he be the boss in a lot of stuff, I still struggle with it right now, believe me. It's not easy taking the most controlling human being on the planet and telling her, "You have to ask your husband what he thinks."

WHAT????? I'm Star Jones, I usually make all the decisions, what do I care what he thinks?

I care. And I anoint him my priest, my prophet, and my king. He's my advocate. I really and truly am *his* advocate. And by the time I was ready to marry him, that's what I wanted: a partner in marriage but a man strong enough to take the lead.

Not everything's all his call. I set the tone for this family—how we're perceived; in many ways, I'm the hedge of protection for us. And listen—sometimes he makes me angry. He can be a big old baby. He can be selfish. He can sulk, and I'm not used to that. But I always go back to "He's the man of my dreams, the man I want in my life long term, and I would rather fight with him than make love to anyone else."

And like me or not for it, that's the transparent me.

Celebration

This one's simple. Be excited about yourselves. You're not allowed to be arrogant, but you can definitely feel self-assured—you've done it, you've found each other, and that's worthy of celebration! So, we honor each other, celebrate our love every waking moment. When I'm all dressed up and ready to walk out the door, Al will say to me in the quietest, sexiest voice, "Let 'em have it, Ms. Jones." You know what that does for me?

"Baby, you are the Man," I'll answer.

"Thank you, baby," he says.

Later on that evening, when we meet again at home, I'll say, "Babe, did you make any money today?"

And he'll say, "Yeah, I think I might have made a little bit of money."

And I say, "Did you go buy your wife something? Because your wife likes pretty things."

And he'll say, "I know my wife likes pretty things. Didn't I give you that big old diamond ring?"

And I'll say, "Oooh, that was last year."

So—we toast each other with humor and appreciation and, yes, with enormous respect. That's my kind of morality.

What's *Not* Morality?

Funny thing: once I asked a guy who was very interested in dating one of my friends, "Do you have a girlfriend?"

"No, that ain't me right now," he answered.

It was a little too hemming and hawing of an answer, so I became the prosecutor and asked what I like to think is the ultimate follow-up question in this situation: "Well, is there anybody out there in the world who *thinks* she's your girlfriend?"

And the guy said after a little more hemming and hawing, "Well, there be a couple of them."

"Well, I'll be doggoned," I answered.

It was my first clue that this guy was not for my friend. He was never going to have a moral relationship, neither with her, nor with anyone probably. Nor will the guy who takes you to church on Sunday and tries to hit it on Monday.

We want to be free to do everything we want anytime we want to do it, and nobody seems to want to pass judgment or even say, "But you know what? That's wrong. It doesn't make me comfortable. It's wrong to sleep around even if it feels good. And if everyone else does it and you use contraceptives so no one will get hurt, it's still just wrong."

Lots of things don't make me comfortable. It doesn't make me comfortable for someone to say that a woman who's a teacher can have a sexual relationship with a child, and seven or eight years later, because the child is eighteen, let's celebrate their marriage. That's wrong. That's immoral.

Do you also have serious issues with making jokes about Michael Jackson and the young boys who sleep at his house? Listen—Michael may have the purest heart in the world, and he may be telling the truth about the innocence of his relationships with boys, and he may mean it that only friendship is in his heart. But that's not what's in everyone else's heart who invites young boys to a sleepover. So Michael has to ask himself if it is right to give a child a false sense of how the rest of the world acts. When you're forty-eight years old and say to a child of nine who's sharing your intimate space that "there are no boundaries between adults and kids," that isn't going to benefit the child in the long run—even if Michael never laid a hand on those boys. Children are not short adults. And the mother has to ask herself whether it was right for her to allow her boy to share the intimate space of an adult, even if she *knew* the adult had the purest intentions. What happened to no? What happened to, "It's no because I'm the momma? I'm the momma and you're not."

What's acceptable to us today probably starts with society's saying, everything goes.

It follows that if you're talking sex and dating, it's not acceptable, it's not moral for a date to refer to a woman—even in jest—as a *bitch* or a *ho*. It's not acceptable for any woman to accept that treatment. Your morals . . . your decisions. I'm just asking.

Passion

Let me say a few words about passion, before I stop talking about sex and dating in a moral relationship. My man—he's passionate. He was when we were dating, and he never stopped. But passion has to be something more than sex. You can have a passion for growing roses, for painting, for exuberance in life.

Al is passionate about some textures—he loves the feel of cashmere. First Christmas, my mother bought him a gray cashmere sweater out of the blue, she didn't know about his passion. He loves that sweater more than any other article of clothing, and whenever he's contemplating something or something's just not right, Al puts on that sweater and his pajama bottoms, and it's like a cocoon for him. So, passion, maybe, is finding the thing the other loves and being willing to give it to him. And passion is being each other's cheerleader.

I'm so passionate about being in his presence that I have to work real hard at not smothering him. I'm passionate about humor—and Al gives it to me. At one point, last week, I was talk, talk, talking, duh duh duh duh, telling him everything that my head held, talkingtalkingtalking, and Al was lying on the bed, and after I talked for a solid fourteen minutes, he quietly said, "Oh my God—I married a woman who talks more than my mother." I couldn't stop laughing for ten minutes. That's a kind of passion.

And once, when we were having a little argument about six weeks before the wedding, I gave him the opportunity to back out, and he said, "How am I going to back out of this wedding when half my family is carrying your veil?"

I mean—you gotta love a guy who makes you laugh.

So, all kinds of passion lie in our lives, and one of the reasons I think it's so powerful is that we proved to each other before our marriage that we could wait for sex, that there was lots of other good stuff besides sex, that we excite each other in a hundred different ways, and that we, together, can distinguish the difference between right and wrong.

Of all things, we find *huge* passion in getting dressed up for each other and going out to dinner. We like to make sure the other looks really good, and then we'll wrap our arms around each other. And he'll say, "Let 'em have it, Ms. Jones."

And I'll say, "Oooooh, baby, you're lookin' good."

Yep, there is someone better than Prince Charming.

Part Three

Be All You Can Be, Spiritually

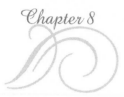

Chapter 8

Stop and Say Thank You

*Spiritual love is a position of standing with one hand extended
into the universe and one hand extended into the world,
letting ourselves be a conduit for passing energy.*

CHRISTINA BALDWIN, EDUCATOR

Sometimes, I need a reminder that God uses other people to send me messages.

Sometimes, I need a reminder that God is there, watching.

Recently, I had a whole lot of stuff that was weighing heavy on my spirit. In the space of one week, I had to do an enormous amount of work, give a speech in Chicago, and fly down to Florida to host an event. My emotional state was very fragile and not least of all because my husband wasn't falling all over me with sympathy. I called him from Florida, and I really lit into him.

"You're not comforting me the way I need to be comforted," I said to him.

"Because I won't crawl into bed with you and allow you to wallow?" he asked.

"Because I think you need to take responsibility for the decisions you make about your life and career?" he asked. "That's not providing comfort. That's babysitting. I'm not that husband. You don't need that from me."

He was right. He'd given me a reality check instead of the babying I was pleading for. But frankly, at the moment I couldn't see that reality check. I was mightily pissed.

So, there I am in Florida, chewing the ear off my girlfriend Jaci, who'd flown down to keep me company. I've done the hosting, and we've done the spa, and we've done the pool, and we're doing the beach—and I'm still feeling pretty mad at Al. Jaci's reading *O: The Oprah Magazine,* which features a little take-away booklet that month. All of a sudden, Jaci says, "I need to share something with you, Star."

Jaci never says "You better listen to this," or "Here's a lesson for you;" right now, she just says she wants to share something that moved her in Oprah's booklet.

And Jaci starts to read me something Oprah's written, describing how she was crying one day because people were being so mean and nasty to her. The people had made up terrible lies and were accusing her of awful stuff, and Oprah was telling all this to Dr. Maya Angelou, the wonderful poet. All of a sudden, in the middle of Oprah's whining and moaning, Dr. Angelou turned to her and firmly said, "Stop—and say thank you, Oprah."

And Oprah looked at Dr. Angelou, amazed, and said, "What do you mean, stop and say thank you? This is horrible for me."

And Maya Angelou spoke hard into Oprah's spirit and said, "If you don't stop and say thank you, I'm not talking to you anymore."

I took a deep breath, stopped, and in my heart, thanked Dr. Angelou. I got it. Then, I turned to Jaci and thanked her. Then, I thanked God. I literally felt God smile right then. It was as if my whole funk about Al had lifted. This is why:

I strongly believe that there are some people who are God-used in life and some people who are God-sent. Al is God-sent to me, okay? Jaci, right then, was God-used just as Maya Angelou was God-used for Oprah. God sometimes uses somebody to convey a message and the message was, Star—I want you to think really long and hard about what has happened in your life.

I thought about how incredibly lucky I was that I could afford to help my family out financially. I thought about how deeply beautiful my life is—the travel I can do, the people who love me, the fun I have in my career, the fascinating friends I have, the good health of those in my closest circles. I thought about how blessed I was to find Al Reynolds, that sweet man. Fact is, I've been able to have a life that most little girls born low-income and black could only dream of.

My dreams, they got me in a whole heap of trouble when planning the "Wedding of My Dreams." And the really interesting thing is . . . I wouldn't change one thing. As I thought about Dr. Angelou's advice, I remember the pain I felt from the media attacks over my completely over-the-top wedding. Al used to say, you don't want a wedding, baby, you want a parade . . . and he was right. But not for the reasons that most people thought.

You know that I come from people who are the salt of the earth. They have earned every dollar they have and still struggle for each and every one. We were not poor, because we knew where every meal was coming from, but *privileged* was not a word in any of our vocabularies. As I planned that over-the-top, parade of a wedding, I thought about what it would mean, not just to me but to my family and my friends. My grandfather is eighty-nine years old. That means as a black man he has lived through Jim Crow, segregation, lynchings, water hoses, separate water fountains, unwelcoming lunch counters, and young white boys calling him "Clyde" when he deserved the respect of being called "Mr. Bennett." He has lived to see his children all attend college and was in the room when his eldest granddaughter, Star, graduated from law school. And on November 13, 2004, he also lived long enough to watch that same granddaughter close a section of Park Avenue as she got married in one of the most beautiful sanctuaries in the world, and—also for her wedding day—close the entire lobby of the greatest hotel in the world, the Waldorf-Astoria. Because of the blessings I have been given, I got to take my grandfather and my eighty-six-year-old grandmother shopping in Saks Fifth Avenue and buy for her her first designer evening gown. I look back on the photos of my grandfather being escorted from his very own suite in that hotel to the front of St. Bartholomew's Church to sit next to Hillary Clinton, a U.S. senator, the former first lady of the United States of America (and possibly the first woman to be the president) and I cry tears of joy. Whatever they have to throw at me can't begin to erase the blessings of what I've been able to do for my family because of this public life.

So, I stopped and said thank you.

And it also came to me how lucky I was to have this man who cared so much about me he wouldn't feed me platitudes. I realized that it's okay to be annoyed with someone and share that when you're dating and certainly after you're married because then you're really communicating. It's not all hearts and flowers and running toward each other in slow motion. I stopped and said thank you.

So, Sunday, I walk into the house after my trip. Now, Al doesn't know I've had this epiphany. He doesn't know that Jaci, the God-used one, had brought me a spiritual knowing. So, I walk into my house, and on the table was a candle, my favorite oatmeal raisin cookie, a little bowl of my favorite barbecue potato chips, and a book called *The Purpose-Driven Life* opened to a highlighted passage that talks about how families grow through stages, and some of them are difficult, and how at any moment, God has you at a stage for a reason.

There was also a hand-created note. Al had cut a ring of flowers from a magazine and laid it down on a piece of construction paper. Inside the ring was written,

I love you. And this is just one stage. Okay?
Al

And next to the note is a little happy face.

Yeah—Jaci was God-used. Yes, I had the epiphany. But the God-sent one came through in a pinch.

Much Is Required

The Bible tells us that to whom much is given, much is required. Now, you can interpret that any way you wish, but now, when I embrace the fact that God has given me so much, I know that means I am *required,* I have a responsibility not only to give back to those who have less but to stop and say thank you to God. And for me, that's spirituality.

I've been brought up in an atmosphere of religion and godliness, but when I was readying myself to meet my soul mate, I knew I had to delve even deeper into spiritual matters. I had the feeling that much more than I was giving was required of me, and it was deeply important that the man for whom I was searching would feel the same way.

Let's talk for a second about that word—religion. Lately, it seems that religion has taken on the mantra of being exclusive rather than inclusive. Being Christian for me means walking in Christ's steps—not being judgmental of others who don't buy into my religion. Being spiritually fulfilled is the same as being religiously fulfilled—and anyone, no matter her faith, can find this comforting spirituality. It's just as available to someone who has very little in her life, as well as to someone who's got the whole world at her fingertips. And if you want to change your life by finding someone to share it with you, it's my feeling that a spiritual balance, along with physical and emotional health, must also be yours.

It's fascinating to note that according to a 2005 *Newsweek* poll and cover story, the vast majority of Americans (88 percent) describe themselves as either spiritual or religious when only a generation ago, a 1966 cover story in *Time* magazine asked, "Is God Dead?" Today, everywhere, says *Newsweek,* is a "flowering of spirituality: in the hollering, swooning, foot-stomping services of the new wave of Pentecostals; in Catholic churches where worshippers contemplate the Eucharist; among Jews who are seeking God in the mystical thickets of Kabbalah . . ."; in Buddhism, in Islam—everywhere. Americans are seeking to experience God in their lives, are seeking to be, as one person put it, grounded in "transformative experience."

Doesn't surprise me. If you are spiritually weak, nothing else matters—I feel that as surely as I know my own name. The thought of approaching life as if there are no ramifications to actions, in my opinion, is what has taken culture down a wayward path and why we're having such trouble in this world right now. There needs to be an unjudgmental but moral standard in politics, and in relationships, as well—in the way parents and children relate to one another, in the way countries relate to one another, men relate to women, employers relate to employees, and definitely how lovers relate to each other. It seems to be that, along with giving personal comfort to us, spiritual strength also helps provide the foundation for that kind of moral standard.

My covenant with God is unshakable: There is nothing else I know in this world that is one hundred percent reliable, dependable, and consistent, now and until the end of time. If the same is true for you, if spirituality is important to you, you must seek a mate who also makes it important in his life—that's what will make you equally yoked. If you're a sports fan, you generally seek out somebody who's a sports fan. If you like art movies, you tend to seek out people who like art movies. If you're a NASCAR fan, and you want to put on those jumpsuits with all that stuff on them, then you'll probably look for a man or woman in an orange jumpsuit just like you. Now, if you spend that kind of effort for your extracurricular activities, why wouldn't you seek out a man who has a gentle, spiritual heart? The thing that holds everything together is my spirituality. It's what's inside me.

Stop for a moment and assess your own sense of spirituality. What's inside *you*?

WHAT'S YOUR SPIRITUAL TYPE?

There are no right or wrong answers in this quiz, no judgments from me or anyone else about whether you're correct in feeling as you do. Spirituality is such an individual, self-propelled state of consciousness that no one can tell what will provide the most joy and sense of completion for another. This self-assessment exercise merely sets out to determine if you feel complete—or if you are longing for something to fill a certain emptiness.

This exercise is also not geared to determine if you're a good Christian, Jew, Muslim, Buddhist—whatever. Although, as you know, Christ is the center of my life, we're not talking about organized religion here: we're talking about relationship, a sense of the holy, a spiritual knowing that God is real. Do you have it? Do you want it? Can you get it? (Yes to the last question.)

Answer either true or false to the following statements.

1. My awareness or consciousness dies when my body dies.   TRUE   FALSE

2. I know there's other "stuff" out there in the universe, even though I'm not religious.   TRUE   FALSE

3. I think I've experienced ESP (extrasensory perception). TRUE FALSE

**4. I'm not religious, but when I'm in trouble,
I can't help but pray to God.** TRUE FALSE

**5. I can't believe in God, because how could a just God tolerate
terrorists, not to mention children with terrible diseases and
tsunamis.** TRUE FALSE

**6. I think people who claim to be spiritual may be sincere but are
horribly misinformed about the nature of the universe.** TRUE FALSE

**7. I often feel so attuned and connected to nature, and even to
certain people I've just met for the first time.** TRUE FALSE

**8. I often feel empty—I have a hunger that is not appeased
even by chocolate or a great pastrami sandwich.** TRUE FALSE

9. When I feel out of control, I surrender to a larger power. TRUE FALSE

10. When I feel out of control, I seize control back. TRUE FALSE

Now choose the answers that best describe you.

11. Being alone in a silent place, makes me:

A. Very nervous
B. Search inward for answers that elude me
C. Long for the next fun party
D. Search the universe for answers

12. The last time I prayed was:

A. Never
B. Within the past year
C. For a celebrity sighting
D. Yesterday or maybe even an hour ago

continued

13. I usually look for love:

A. In all the wrong places
B. Within my family
C. And find it—and it's invariably, the wrong person
D. In the right places

14. About mystical stuff, I think:

A. It's all hooey.
B. There are no such thing as miracles and a rational explanation for everything.
C. I'm open to new possibilities; I wish someone could prove that other forces existed—but no one ever has, at least to me.
D. There are many extraordinary things that can't be explained by science—even by the head of the department.

15. I believe that God or another spiritual force:

A. Does not exist
B. Is a wish, a dream, an ideal—but not real. I don't think
C. Can intervene in my life—and I know I can prove it
D. Does intervene in my life—and I feel I can prove it

16. I know this is true:

A. I have a sixth sense that often allows me to anticipate when something is going to happen.
B. We only have one time around and we must use it to the fullest.
C. God is real.
D. This is a haphazard world.

17. I believe that what is written in holy books (the Bible, Koran, etc.):

A. Is divinely inspired
B. Are human-created stories passed down through the ages
C. Are meant to be seen as metaphors—not really holy wisdom
D. Are interesting mythology, plain and simple

18. I think that a future mate of mine:

A. Can believe anything he wishes about God; it has no consequence to the happiness of our marriage, even if I believe directly opposite.
B. Ought to feel as spiritually disinclined as I do.
C. Ought to be more practical than spiritual.
D. Ought to believe deeply and have a personal relationship with God, as I do.

19. For me, spirituality means:

A. Zero, zilch, nada.
B. A deep feeling that there's something or someone greater than me out there.
C. Certain people need psychological crutches—and that's fine. I'm just not one of them.
D. A relationship with God.

20. Sometimes, I find myself:

A. Waiting for a miracle or a direction or . . . something.
B. Marveling at places that seem actually sacred—great forests, cathedrals of rocks, snow-covered mountains, the sea.
C. Impatient with those who don't take responsibility for their decisions, but plead for help from God.
D. Looking for meaning in life—but I'm not at all sure it will come from a divine source.

SCORING

1. T=0, F=5
2. T=5, F=0
3. T=5, F=0
4. T=10, F=0
5. T=0, F=5
6. T=0, F=5
7. T=15, F=0
8. T=5, F=0
9. T=15, F=0
10. T=0, F=5

continued

11. A=0, B=10, C=0, D=10

12. A=0, B=5, C=0, D=10

13. A=0, B=5, C=0, D=10

14. A=0, B=0, C=5, D=10

15. A=0, B=5, C=5, D=10

16. A=10, B=2, C=10, D=0

17. A=10, B=0, C=2, D=0

18. A=0, B=0, C=5, D=10

19. A=0, B=10, C=0, D=10

20. A=10, B=5, C=0, D=3

ANALYSIS: Add up your score

If you scored from 0 to 25, you are a Confirmed Skeptic.

When it comes to an awareness of spirituality in yourself or anyone else, you have a prove-it mentality, and for some people, I do understand that's enormously reassuring—knowing that nothing exists unless you can see, taste, touch, hear, or smell it. You're very resistant to any idea of God or another power in the universe, and you're certainly opposed to trying to build spiritual awareness in your heart. You're an existentialist—someone who believes in every individual as a self-determining agent, responsible for his or her choices. Certainly, the religious landscape to you is barren.

Look—I wholly respect your right to skepticism, even though it makes me a little sad to consider what I think you're missing. Do me a favor: be open-minded. Read through the following section anyway. If you come to think there may be the tiniest room for you to develop the tiniest connection to God—then your pal Star feels a whole lot happier. If you read the following and still feel certain there's no room for spirituality in your life, may I advise that you look for a partner who feels the same way (remember, you have to be equally yoked). You know what? You don't have to believe. I'm praying for you anyway.

If you scored from 26 to 91, you're a Spiritual Straddler.

Hey—you just don't know so you straddle and live on both sides of the fence. That makes you able to feel both sides of the issue—both the skeptic's and the believer's.

You very well understand the saying "There are no atheists in foxholes," because when you're in trouble or frightened, you do find yourself praying—to Someone or Something, you're never sure. Nevertheless, you can't figure out what spirituality means. You do feel a strong connection to nature and maybe even something greater than yourself, but you have problems with organized religion. In your experience stuff has happened that can't be scientifically explained, but you have trouble attributing that to a higher presence. Most of all, you can't figure out what's expected of you: how can you pray if you're not sure someone's listening? How do you actually talk to God—if he or she exists? You feel like a moral person, but morality doesn't belong to spirituality. Does it? The best news: you're pretty open-minded and willing to trust your experience if you had a magical spiritual moment. You're waiting.

Did you score from 92 to 148? You're a Spiritual Seeker.

You're almost there because fact is, too many remarkable things have happened to you to throw spirituality out the window. Yes, there's stuff out there—that you now believe, but what and where and how can you find truth? There are dark valleys you've come through, and petty, vindictive, mean-spirited people in your path who have made you distrust a higher being. But then, sometimes you're given a gift of incredible insight and hope, and you are so tempted to believe in some kind of divinity. So, you keep seeking.

Maybe you don't know any technical words to use in prayer, but you strongly feel you've connected with something deep and beautiful, even when you use your own words.

So you keep seeking.

I promise you, sister, you will find.

And I wish for you a love of your life who is also seeking.

Did you score from 149 to 175? You are Deeply Spiritual.

You undoubtedly own a powerful sense that otherworldly forces stronger than you exist. For you, there is truth and comfort in belief in God or other intangible/holy/moral essences. The vital essence of God is with you always. Your nature is metaphysical—highly abstract, subtle, poetical—right? Faith is so important because it helps you cope with hardships and meanness. Sometimes you feel doubt, sure, but it doesn't scare you because in the words of Isaac Bashevis Singer, "Doubt is part of all religion. All the great religious thinkers were doubters." To doubt is to be human.

This is what you believe in: yourself, forgiveness, compassion, joy, and generosity. You're committed to a sacred presence who guides you and takes over with the big decisions when they baffle you. Read on to see how much I share with you.

Chapter 9

The Ultimate Comforter and 9/11

However you scored in your spiritual self-assessment, please, sister, read on. Even some scientist friends who are confirmed skeptics have confided in me that they've had unusual, unexplainable, even mystical experiences or feelings. Has this never happened to you? I'm not trying to proselytize here—you are absolutely entitled to your own nonbeliefs, but if you've read this far, can I just ask you to share my experiences as I prepared myself spiritually for what would be the biggest relationship in my life? It'll make us bond better, friend.

Christ for me is the ultimate comforter. I have known the most amazing relationships with my family and friends; exciting, romantic, and passionate relationships with men, but with all of these people, I've never known the constant peace that my relationship with Christ gives me. It is truly perfect peace.

I've always been a spiritual person because I was raised in a family where we went to church every Sunday, vacation Bible school during the summer, and revival meetings in between. Both my North Carolina grandmothers wouldn't have it any other way. I'm used to getting up and going to Sunday school at nine thirty, to church again for the eleven o'clock service, lunch at the church, then to the three o'clock service or the six o'clock revival. That's church all day, if you're counting. And just so we wouldn't forget what we'd heard all day, the pastor would come to our house for dinner on Sunday to remind us, yet again.

Still, with all that, I don't think it really jelled—what an intimate relationship with God meant—until college, when I got involved in my gospel choir. And then, when I discovered what a lonely place law school can be, I worked even harder at it with my great friend Pastor Kirbyjon Caldwell.

But it really *all* came together for me when I watched that second plane go into the towers on 9/11. I was with my colleagues at *The View* in the makeup room; we were preparing for the morning meeting when the first plane went in. We didn't see the footage immediately—nobody knew what was happening. It looked like a fire—maybe somebody had a little prop plane that got lost and slammed into the towers; you couldn't really read the devastation from the television. But when the second plane hit within minutes, I knew something very bad was happening. Without talking, Jakki Taylor, one of my producers, and my prayer partner and makeup artist, Elena George, and I got up from our chairs in that crowded room, walked into the restroom, and started to pray.

No one had said, "What should we do?" We just knew we had to pray.

Strangely, as we talked about it later, we all agreed that our prayers weren't for one another. We were each praying to God that he would allow us to understand what was going on, that he would tell us that he was in ultimate control. That would give me calm.

God came through.

We knew we had to get home. I had four friends on the show who lived in Jersey, Queens, and the Bronx, and we heard that every tunnel and bridge had been shut down, so because I could get home, I ended up having those four women come to stay with me in my Manhattan apartment. We stood on my terrace, and we looked toward the smoke. It had been the most beautiful day, and when those towers went, it was just gorgeous out, and then—only that oily, awful black smoke.

Want to know what perfect peace is? Over the next couple of weeks, I remember praying constantly for understanding, and where I couldn't understand, for faith. I had to travel a lot on planes, and I did not feel scared—I did not feel scared once.

That's what perfect peace is. Not feeling scared in scary moments. I wasn't afraid of terrorists on my planes or of what could happen next in the world. I was establishing a real relationship with God, and that was eternal and much stronger than terrorists. That's why I call my spirituality the ultimate comfort.

But Could It Last?

Oh yes. There are days when as a woman, your parents don't understand, your family gets on your nerves, your friends have their own priorities, the boyfriend is not acting right, you're just not happy. After 9/11, prayer never failed to help me find happiness in other places. And I felt that the happier I was with God, the happier God was with me.

Instead of looking outward for the blessings that I hoped were coming to me, I started trying to bless other people. Doing something for others made me feel even more blessed. Everyone has to find her own fountain of calmness and peace, and that fountain doesn't have to be an organized religion, but it should include the universal truths that appear in every religion.

Now, I know this: I could have made it alone, I'm a strong woman, but I would not feel complete without Al in my life. He's made me better. I was pretty cool before him, but I'm even better now. That's the way I feel about my relationship with God. I'm better because of my relationship with God—smarter, stronger, more centered, and more solid. I'm nicer. I care more about people, I give and get the blessings, and then, I can get through the crap. And I don't have to tell you, there can be some mean stuff in your life—people have tragedies, you lose children, the first time you bury somebody close to you: you need a deep well into which you can dip for comfort.

How Would You Know That the Ultimate Comforter Was Missing from Your Life?

What would be a sign? An emptiness, that would be your best sign. A feeling of being incomplete or hungry no matter how much you have or how heartily you've eaten. If someone would say to you, "Vanda, you've published twenty books, made five blockbuster movies, and are a mega millionaire, how do you feel?" And the answer would be, "Empty—I feel empty," that's a good clue that something grand and spiritual is missing from your life.

You feel empty when you're hungry because you get a stomachache or a headache, and so, you go looking for food. But if you eat and you're hungry again right away, there's probably something else you need besides food to fill that hunger. When I was overeating, I would gorge to get rid of the craving, but I now know the hunger was not for food, it was for completion. Once I started getting healthy, I didn't have that kind of emptiness. So, even though I thought I had a wonderful relationship with God, I had to deepen that connection.

Relationship, Not Religion

I'm Protestant but nondenominational. I don't need to be a Baptist or a Methodist. My relationship is with Jesus Christ—that's all I need. One of the most important things I did when working on my relationship with God was to search for relationship, not religion. The word *religion* often makes people uncomfortable because people tend to claim it for their own purposes that have nothing to do with God or spiritual comfort. Some misguided fundamentalist Muslims claimed religion as the reason they flew their planes into the World Trade Center, but any true Muslim will tell you that was a truly antireligious, ungodly deed. What's uncomfortable for me is living in a world where there is so much hypocrisy masquerading as religion, where some "religious" person can stand in a pulpit on Sunday, proselytize on morality, and sexually assault a child on Monday. Hypocrisy is when a prominent minister has an affair outside of his marriage, and even though I know that anyone can be redeemed, hearing about religious hypocrisy still makes people weary of religion.

Okay—you're allowed to be weary of religion, but don't be weary of a relationship with God. The ability to pray and to recognize that you don't know everything and that you need some help—that's relationship.

As I explored my spirituality and my deepening connection with Christ, I recognized that I couldn't live my life without God. Personally, I also understood I couldn't live my life without a human relationship that had its strength in spirituality. I know that many women don't feel the same way: they're wonderfully independent and choose to live their lives unattached to a partner. That's fine, of course. But it's different for me. Although the ultimate relationship was with God, I needed a man to help me feel fulfilled and complete, who felt the same way I did about God.

So I did my Bible studies, I went to services and trying to understand more, I consciously tried to do more things for other people, not just for me. It's funny—on *The View,* Madonna said she started writing children's books because her kaballah teacher told her exactly that: "Why don't you do something that's not for you." Now, I think that's the essence of the spiritual woman—to love her neighbor as she loves herself.

I stopped focusing on Star. I got out of the house and volunteered in soup kitchens. Because I'm a fashion plate and love clothes, I went down to an organization called Dress for Success and helped put clothes on the backs of women who've never owned a workplace suit. A friend of mine, also working on developing her relationship with God, loves to dance, and so she used to go to an assisted living facility to teach seniors how to boogie. I started feeling so much better about Star Jones.

I used to tell my mother, "I'm exhausted, tired, I need to rest." Once, having enough, she said to me, "Star, exhausted is raising two children as a single woman, working two jobs, and trying to stay off public assistance. That's exhausted; I don't want to hear that you're exhausted."

When I stopped whining and started doing for others, exhaustion flew out the window. I didn't know it then, but I really was on the last leg of my journey to prepare myself physically, emotionally, and spiritually to meet my life partner.

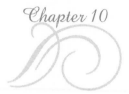

Chapter 10

Bless This Table

Then, I met him. You already heard that story.

So, now Al's in the picture. We met, fell in love, and got engaged in three months. Sure, we talked about our commitment to God. But how did I really know we were on the same page, spiritually? I found out.

He asked me to go to his uncle's funeral with him and his family only three weeks into our relationship. I went down to Horsepasture, Virginia—that's where Al's from—and I thought this would be a good time to check out each other's roots because my grandparents lived very close, and we could go to see them afterward. I stood with Al at the funeral, and afterward, we went back to his mom's house. Al had been telling his mother, "Oh, I met this great girl, and, Mom, she's the one, she's the one, she's the one."

Miss Ada—that's what I call his mom—had been watching me on television, getting a chuckle out of me on *The View,* but frankly, she had her doubts. I was a pretty public person, and they were good, quiet, religious people. After the funeral, Al's mom asked him and two of his brothers to come home with her to put up a mailbox. In the culture of many southern families, no matter who their men are, no matter who their guests are, the mother says put up a mailbox, you put a mailbox up. And of course, Al took on his customary role as supervisor.

Afterward, Al comes in, and the supervisor's wiped out because he had been working and traveling all week. And Miss Ada, who was cooking in her kitchen, and I, sitting in the family room, started to talk. Their family room adjoins the kitchen so you can talk right through the two rooms. While the pot was doing what it was doing in the kitchen, Miss Ada came out to sit on a stool next to me on the settee. Then Al came in and lay down on the settee next to me and put his head right down in my lap—with his mom sitting there.

So, next thing I know, absentmindedly I'm stroking his head, which is one of his favorite things, and he falls asleep on my lap. There we were—just the three of us, one of us comatose, and his mother says to me, "Is this all real?"

And I say, "Absolutely."

And she says, "How will you know what to do when all this fun and frivolity fades? What will you do then?"

And I say to her, "That's when we'll start praying."

Later, Miss Ada told me she fell in love with me at that moment. That moment right there. She knew how truly I meant it. And then, Miss Ada and I had a conversation about how none of this would ever work or be worth it if Al and I were not united in our faith. I knew that it would be tough for us, and that we'd be the subject of tremendous scrutiny because I'm a television personality, and it's just the nature of celebrity for others to go rag on visible people. We live in an age where paparazzi run their cars into a young Lindsay Lohan's car just so they can get a photograph. We live in a world where a man thinks it's funny to squirt water in Tom Cruise's face (thank God it wasn't acid or urine). We live in that world now, so both Miss Ada and I knew it would be tough for Al and his family.

Later, Al told his family, "I know this feels fast moving, but it's clear to us that we're moving toward permanence. I want you to know that we're very serious, and she's very important to me. I love her, and there will be lots of things said in the media, and I'm going to need you all."

Miss Ada was okay with that. She'd seen my heart. And then, we prayed as a family.

We held hands and made a circle. It's typical of both our families to pray that way—the most natural thing in the world. I needed to be with a man for whom it would be natural. You know what? I was sorry his uncle died, but before I really committed to Al, I had to go into his house in his small town, and before we had a meal, I had to see his family bless the table. I knew then, that when Al and I sat down at a meal in a restaurant, it wouldn't be uncomfortable for him if I reached for his hand and said, "Let's bless the food." I knew when I made dinner at our own home on a Sunday or a Friday or whenever and I said, "Babe, bless the table," he'd know what I meant.

You just need to know that I've spent as much time focused on his relationship with God as I did with all the other silly things that women think about like, Can this boy dress? Am I going to have to start from scratch with him because if he doesn't know how to wear his jeans, like if he wears them too tight, I would *not* like that, okay? Women often spend time on that silliness, especially me: Does he know how to wear his hair? Does he wear too much jewelry? I can't stand a man who smells too much, but I like a little cologne. So, you spend all that time on the superficial. You don't spend any time on the stuff that's really going to get you through when it's funky.

Can he bless his table? If Al could bless his table, we'd be all right.

Then, we left there and went to my grandparents all in the same weekend. We went out to dinner together, we sat in my grandparents' house, and my grandfather, who doesn't say an awful lot because he's now eighty-nine, sat there, watching Al. My grandmother talked to Al. And Al blessed my family's table, and we prayed before dinner, and we prayed before we got on the plane.

And we were a family yoked in spirituality.

Some Amazing Statistics

The MacArthur Foundation in a recent study found that seven out of ten Americans say they're religious and they consider spirituality to be an important part of their lives, *but* only about half of all Americans attend services—and even those go less often than once a month. The same study also says that one in three people have left the religion of their birth.

I feel that one of my personal purposes in life is to show the glory of the satisfied and spiritual life. People can manifest such a life in different ways, but I get to be on television and expose issues I think are wrong, I get to be a philanthropist, and I get to write this book and, I hope, help people looking for love in all the wrong places. It's all fun stuff, but in the end, I hope that my personal spirituality encourages me to be nice to people, to give back to my community, to care what others think (I never did before), and not to be arrogant. Most of all, I want my life to show thanks and worship of God—I'm the one he placed in this blessed position, and I want to stop and say thank you.

So, how do you come to spirituality if you've never been there before?

Chapter 11

How Do You Talk to God?

The absolutes or truisms that you've been reading throughout this book have always worked for me in all aspects of my life. But as I build my relationship with God, there are some that transcend all others. They're pure and positive ways to find spirituality, and I know not to doubt them. When I want to talk to God, they're my absolutes and they help me find the way.

Spiritual Absolutes

When pride enters, wisdom is corrupted.

To walk humbly with God is to be quick to repent, quick to forgive, and quick to remain teachable.

Talent can take you places where character cannot sustain you.

The power to define is the power to validate, and you don't give that power to anyone other than God.

continued

Your conscience either accuses you or excuses you.

Most people live by preference. God teaches us to live by conviction.

A faithful person also makes mistakes—
but is quick to repent when she does.

How else can you find your way to God? These work for me:

A Quiet Mind

It's the best way to find your way to him. The poet Kahlil Gibran says we speak when we feel uncomfortable with the silence of our minds—"You talk when you cease to be at peace with your thoughts." For me, I hear and talk best to God when my mind is quiet. Then, I hear the silence of the still, small voice within me, the silence of strength and contemplation, the silence of the spirit. My grandma used to sing an old spiritual called "Blessed Quietness."

Blessed quietness, holy quietness,
What assurance in my soul,
On the stormy sea, Jesus speaks to me,
And the billows cease to roll.

I think that regularly, we have to still the static, still the news, the laughter, the air conditioners, the traffic, the phones, even occasionally still *The View* to make the blessed quiet we need to hear God's voice. We have to carve out time every week for solitude, meditation, prayer, and soul searching for private talks with God.

Be quiet and listen, and the spirit will work through your mind. Don't expect Moses' experience of God's booming voice giving him the Ten Commandments. It is a calmer, soundless voice you'll hear. And don't just speak to God; let God speak to you. Why is it that we think we always have to be in control?

Sometimes you just need to shut up. Shut up and listen for a minute. Your brain, your mind, your heart, it all talks to you.

Ever dated someone you know is no good for you? When you go in that quiet place by yourself, and the door is closed, and you shut everything down, every single thing that has been bothering you bubbles right to the surface. You don't need anybody to tell you to make him history, that no-good guy. You don't. But, see—that's God talking to you.

One day, I talked about this on television. It was actually on the day of my bridal shower. I explained that I was no longer allowing anything mean-spirited to come into my ears or to have an impact on my psyche because it was my job to break up Satan's airwaves. It's like you're listening to a sweet radio station, and you're jamming to your song, and your fingers are popping, and all of a sudden static just messes it all up. That's Satan trying to mess you up so you won't hear God's voice.

Satan?

You bet—Satan. I definitely think you can't believe in God without believing that there's evil. There are people who will do everything in their power to rob you of your blessing. I live this day by day. I know there are people out there who are unhappy with themselves, and so their mission is to make you unhappy, too. Al and I were really tested during our engagement period. One day we would read that Al was out gallivanting with a bunch of women. The next day, we'd read a story questioning his sexuality.

I remember my husband saying to me, "Baby—what am I today?" And me answering, "Just who you were yesterday, baby." The attacks on the nature of our relationship never bothered me a bit because I knew this man. But attacks on me, saying I was nasty or discourteous—those hurt so because I could not challenge the rumormongers. Al would give me strength one day, and I'd give him strength the next, and we prayed every morning and every evening, and we still do.

But you know what, even if there's Satan static in your life, you bring in Nancy Wilson and her rendition of "What a Difference a Day Makes," and it doesn't matter what kind of nasty stuff is going on, she makes it better. Doesn't have to be an old-time spiritual to be a spiritual.

". . . twenty-four little hours, brought the sun and the flowers, where there used to be rain."

Oh, Nancy. I stop and give thanks for Nancy.

Rituals

Can I say a few words about ritual? You know religion is filled with ritual—the sprinkling of the holy water, the incense, the candles, the prayer rugs, the communion. I think in life we should make up our own rituals; they hold magic, they bring us quiet and calm so we can hear the voice of God. Again, this has nothing to do with religion and everything to do with a relationship with God.

I've got one ritual I've never changed for years. When I get on a plane, I need to quiet myself, I need to find comfort in spirituality. So, I pray the same prayer—it always works. And now Al prays it with me. I say, "God, we're about to fly in your sky. Please send down your angels to safely guide us on their wings to our destination."

I made it up, and that visual gets us through a fourteen-hour flight. You ask God to do you a favor and send down his protectors, his angels, to get onto this giant bird and glide you down safely. I've got more faith in God's angels than I do in that plane.

Another ritual: Al and I like to not end a conversation mean—even if we're annoyed with each other. We talk until we can get to a point where we can end it where we've said something pleasant to each other. You don't want to end it mean. You don't.

And my shower ritual. That's private time with God in the morning. Just me and him and that soothing water cascading down. And lately I notice Al does the same thing. I hear him talking to God in his shower.

We also have a phone ritual. If, say, Al has a big presentation in the morning, I know we'll hold hands and pray at the house before we both leave, but the ritual isn't complete until Al calls me on the phone to say, "Hey, I'm about to go into the meeting." That's my cue to say something like, "Father God, bless this meeting, and we want to thank you for our relationship and the fact we can rely on each other through you. We know Al is going to use every bit of his talent, intelligence, heart, and spirit you've given him because all this is done for your glory."

And if Al doesn't score at the meeting? That means we're on to the next great thing God has planned for us. We walk the path together. It's what God wants.

Create your own rituals. They're little ceremonies, sweet observances that you do over and over. They bring peace and a sense of mystical other worldliness.

Laughing

Humor is an absolute in my life, and it has everything to do with my personal brand of spirituality. God's not so serious that you have to be so proper in his presence. Sometimes, when I have to do something hard in God's name, I'll say to Al, "Woo! Jesus is no joke!" Then, sometimes I'll hear a sermon, and within an hour, I will hear a song about exactly the same thing. I then know what God wants me to do. I laugh to myself, thinking, "God, if you wanted me to know it, just tell me. You didn't have to smack me in the head, okay?"

But sometimes, yes, he does have to smack me in the head, because I'm not listening. So, when you hear a message being broadcast to you every which way, through a song, through a newspaper headline, through a whispered voice, just say out loud, "Oh, *that's* what you wanted!"

Sometimes, you know, if you don't deal with whatever issues are going on in your life privately, God will have to deal with them publicly. It's the only way he can get your attention.

Stacked

Albert Einstein once said, there are two ways to live your life: one, as if nothing is a miracle, and the other is as if everything is a miracle. Here's an absolute: in my life, everything is a miracle and planned by the miracle maker. My pastor once said that nothing that God does is by happenstance. It is all according to a plan and for a purpose. If you walk down a street, said Pastor Bernard, and you see a bunch of change strewn across the sidewalk, your first thought is, "Oh my God, somebody dropped their money out their pocket." But if you walked down the street and saw quarters stacked up in a stack, you'd say, "Somebody put those quarters there."

As I look at my world and how things are in my life, somebody put those quarters there. Somebody stacked 'em up. Somebody put those quarters down for me to retrieve. There are no accidents. There's a reason behind each and every thing. Think about my life.

I was born to a single mother in a town in North Carolina. I had two sets of grandparents who decided "our baby's not gonna want for anything, so we're gonna take care of her and between the two sets of grandparents, we'll make sure she has everything she needs. My biological father's sister, my Aunt Shirley, happened to be an educator, so I learned to read before most children. I started school earlier than most children, skipped the second grade, went straight from the first grade to the third grade. Moved to New Jersey, lived in a housing project while my mom struggled with low income. My mother instilled pride and purpose into my life as a little girl because as a little girl, *she* climbed her way out of poverty, became a social worker, helping others do the same thing. My mother started directing one of the relief agencies that she used to benefit from, and I graduated from high school. I won every community-based scholarship that was available to win so I could pay for school—every one except the Jewish one, and I couldn't win that because I wasn't Jewish. My mother didn't say, "Pick a community college. Pick a local school." My mother said, "Pick the best school you want, we'll figure out how to pay for it." I worked throughout college every single day, work-study job for the first two months because that's what you get. Then, I taught myself how to increase my typing speed, took myself down to the Brookings Institution, and got one of those part-time typist jobs, typed 90 words per minute, so I went from a work-study job making $4 an hour to making $10 an hour as a freshman. Worked my way through college. Applied to law school. Worked my way through law school. Came out of law school owing $70,000 in student loans—$70,000! Took my dream job that paid very little money—$22,500 a year as an assistant district attorney. That's the job I wanted. I didn't think about the fact that I could have gotten one of these law firm jobs that paid $75,000 which would pay back some of those loans. I took my dream job because that's the job I thought could help me give the most back. Spent more than I earned (that shopping thing again). Went into terrible debt. I had the credit collection agencies calling me, and me saying, "You know, Ms. Jones, she don't live here no more"—that kind of thing. It was so embarrassing. Got my wages garnished as an assistant district attorney, but I plugged along. And I plugged along. I was kicking butt in the courtroom, and somehow, some way, somebody saw me do some commentary in the beginning of Court TV. I got a phone call to come and do the first weekend of Court TV, and a young booker from NBC said to someone important, "You know, she's special." The Important One called, brought me on the *Today* show, and six weeks later, I became a national news correspondent, for NBC News, for the *Today* show and for *Nightly News with Tom Brokaw*. This little girl from a small town in North Carolina. Within a year, I'd paid those loans back.

Now, you tell me that somebody hasn't stacked those quarters up for me.

That change was not just dropped there, momma.

Reflect God's Shining Face

"The Lord makes his face to shine upon you," and I think that we have to be mirrors of God's shining face, and it is my job as a reflector to send that radiance right back to you, okay? That's an absolute, a truism. It's what I should do.

But I don't—not always, anyway. Every time I don't do it is when I disappoint God and when I do a disservice to him.

Recently, I really forgot that God is reflected in everything I do.

There is a radio host, very popular with a certain segment of society, who has been vicious to me for several years straight. I don't think there is a word in the dictionary that could adequately describe what nasty is when it comes to his comments. He might think they're funny. He might just mean to appeal to his audience, but his remarks about me are the basest, most vulgar examples of immorality, intolerance, and viciousness that I can imagine. It's been relentless. He makes my heart hurt. But never once did I address his comments directly.

Never once until I found myself baited on television one day, and I fell into a trap.

We were having a conversation on the show about censorship and whether or not this radio personality's comments should be censored by the FCC. Somehow, I allowed my emotional self to respond instead of that purpose-driven woman I know I am.

What did I say? I said there were certain people that quite frankly, didn't deserve to have their comments heard, and I thought his remarks didn't fall within the purview of free speech. But then, instead of just making my opinion known, I went very personal.

"I couldn't care less if the vultures ate upon his body," I commented.

Okay—it wasn't very pithy and it sure was mean. Actually, what I said was so intense and mean-spirited, I gotta tell you, immediately thereafter, *I felt so good.* I felt wonderful. I felt it's about doggone time. And I got e-mail from people saying, "It's about time." My girlfriends called me saying, "It's about time." Oh my gosh. I came home, and I bragged to Al, "Baby, this is what I did, and da da da da da," and his response to me was, "Does it make you feel better?"

"Yes, it makes me feel better," I shot back.

I went to sleep that night and I did not sleep at all—not one wink of sleep the entire night. I felt the presence of the Holy Spirit fighting with me that entire night because your conscience either excuses you or accuses you, and my conscience was not excusing me that night. Next morning, I got up and confessed on national television that I had allowed somebody to take me away from the person I know I am, and no matter how vicious somebody is to me, it is my job to reflect God's shining face. And I hadn't.

I made a mistake. Look, I know that I am not perfect. I know that I say and do things that cause God to shake his head, but I always try. On that day, I didn't try. I promised myself that I would not do that ever again. And I haven't.

But now I'm free from that man's despicable arrows. Like me, don't like me, say mean things, don't say mean things—I don't care because it doesn't have an impact on my spirit anymore. I'm past it. And you know what? Because I live in a free country, and the radio host needs to accept my personal choices, I now firmly believe I also need to accept that man's choice to belittle me. And as much as I despise him, if someone tried to stop his freedom of speech, I'd be out there marching for his right to speak. He's vulgar, he's mean, but he's American.

So that's how you get your mirror to reflect God's shining face.

No one ever said it would be easy.

Relationships

I've been talking to God for a long time now, and we've developed a pattern of conversation; I say *we've* developed because I'm certain God hears, and responds. In fact, my relationship with God is sort of a template for my relationship with everyone else. If I can get it right with God, I sure ought to be able to get it right with anyone I care about. So, I follow the same guidelines I use when I talk to God. I actually have some tenseness with a girlfriend, and our relationship has changed forever.

First of all, I have to be honest with myself and ask myself what I did to cause the friction. The hardest thing in the world is to shine the light on yourself, okay? It's rare that friction is the fault of only one person, so after I assessed my role in the matter, I scheduled some time to talk to my friend—and admitted what *I* did before I addressed the whole issue and how sad it made me feel.

This is sort of how you go to God and ask for forgiveness for something or relief from the tension that's overwhelming. The first thing you do is acknowledge what you did wrong. When you talk to God, you don't start going, "Oh, God, please bless me with this new job." If it's a new job that you are seeking, you say, "God, you know, I have not always done the best with the resources that you have provided me. I've made poor decisions in my finances. I've allowed my desire for pretty things to overcome my desire to take care of my long-term needs, but I finally put myself in such a position that I have gotten my credit in order. I have another opportunity, a second chance, and this is a blessing. Please bless me again and help me to learn from my mistakes."

Same thing with my friend. After I assess what I've done, I go to that friend in the same vein I would go to God asking God's forgiveness. I'll have to say something to her like, "You know, it's clear that our relationship has changed, and

I've asked myself what I've done to add to that change. I'm sorry that I haven't been calling, and I'm sorry that I've put you off, and I'm sorry that I haven't valued what you had to offer to this relationship. And I need you to know that I don't put it all on you. I have to recognize that I had something to do with it, that I, not just you, own our tension. But together, we have to figure out how I can not add to the problem any more and you won't add to the problem—and we can be as we were before."

Most of us pray privately. We can talk to God privately, even without words. But when it comes to other people, you have to get those words out. Okay, call it a conversation, but whatever you call it, you should both kind of pray together that you can restore your friendship. And then, you can move on.

Sometimes, I'm sorry to tell you, moving on means that the relationship is changed, and maybe even over. But change is not bad. Change, based on knowledge and honesty with each other, is like a prayer.

Here's an extraordinary bonus: when you quiet your mind, besides hearing God, you can also hear the needs of others. If you spend all your time whimpering, "I'm bored. My life's not complete. Nobody loves me. I don't have a man," you're whining and nobody loves a whiner. And you are deaf to the suffering around you—a bad thing.

We're all tempted to bemoan our fate, but now when I do that, I force myself to think, "Somebody lost her child in Iraq today. There's a woman down in Aruba searching for her daughter. There's a young black woman from Spartanburg, South Carolina, who's been missing for a year—her parents go to bed every night wondering what happened to their child. Someone's going to bed hungry tonight."

If you shut your mouth for a moment when you feel overwhelmed, you'll find a way to help someone who has a real tragedy. Guess what? That will make you feel immensely better. That's the essence of spirituality.

Forgiveness

*If we practice an eye for an eye, and a tooth for a tooth,
soon the whole world will be blind and toothless.*

MAHATMA GANDHI

The weak never forgive. Forgiveness is an attribute of the strong.

MAHATMA GANDHI

Always forgive your enemies. Nothing annoys them more.

OSCAR WILDE

I believe all of the above. It's important to be able to forgive because holding on to grievances and anger causes grief and frustration. That's absolutely an absolute. Seems to me, though, we don't forgive someone because the person we're forgiving necessarily deserves it. Forgiveness is also not excusing someone or validating his point of view. It's not even a favor you do for someone who's hurt you (so she can do it again). Being able to let the pain of betrayal and misunderstanding go is a gift we give to ourselves—not to the person who's been obnoxious. Forgiving another brings the same blessing we get when God forgives us.

But guess what? You know how they say, "Forgive and forget"? Well, they're wrong. Don't even try to forget—not going to happen, no matter what they tell you. But forgiveness? That's another matter.

Being able to forgive makes us feel generous and powerful. We're no longer victims who've been hurt; now we're aggressively forgiving. We open ourselves up to healing. And it works especially well if we can take some responsibility, some ownership of what happened that was bad.

No question, though, one of the hardest things in the world to do is to forgive. Still, as a Christian, I have to say to myself, "There's nothing anybody did to me any worse than what they did to Christ." So, if he can forgive, so can Star.

The Psalms tell us that Christ's willingness to forgive is universal, and if we expect forgiveness, we must be ready to forgive.

Okay—I can just hear you asking, "So, Star—can you forgive that certain radio personality?"

Already done. Believe it. If I couldn't forgive him, I couldn't do what I do every day. He's absolutely forgiven because now I know he's irrelevant. Somebody who means nothing to me is an easy forgive—he's just not present in my real life, he's not going to take any food off my table. My mama's still gonna live in her house. My friends are still gonna come visit. My dog, Pinky, and I are still gonna fool around. My husband is still gonna come home and say, "Baby, what you got to eat?" every day.

But what happens when someone you deeply care for hurts you? See, if I could no longer trust Al, that would be hard to forgive. I would try, but I can't swear I'd succeed. What if Al did something really bad, like running around with another woman?

I think it would kill my unconditional trust for him.

But you know what? I feel God would help me out with that one. That's why Al and I had so many sessions of premarital counseling before we walked down the aisle, just to be able to recognize that loved ones make mistakes. I'm not telling you that Al has free rein to do something that's a violation of our covenant. But I know that our marriage is strong enough to sustain me from being irreparably crushed by something he says or does.

If he fooled around, nothing would ever be the same, it's true. Our marriage would be changed forever. But the question is, would I be able to live with that change if he were truly sorry? Could I forgive him? Well, I think my spiritual commitment provides me with a comfortable cashmere sweater like Al's that allows me to adapt. If he did something really terrible, it would not be what I hoped or dreamed for, but maybe I could forgive even though I'd never forget.

I sure pray Al uses the same level of commitment to the covenant as I do.

Now, if there were to come a time when the man himself changed, that would be very different. That would disappoint me irrevocably. The man I know wouldn't easily breach his covenant. But he won't. Here's why:

Al's a big old baby. He'd be the first one to tell you, "Nobody knows how to take care of me the way my wife takes care of me. What am I gonna do with those little hoochies out there—they don't even know how I like my shirts."

One night, he traveled all day to get back to me and our home in the Hamptons. I was at a meeting when he arrived, but I'd stopped off earlier to buy him something for dinner. When I got home, he was asleep.

"Baby, I told you to stay up and wait for me," I whispered.

"You were taking too long, Star," he muttered back from a deep dream.

"I got dinner for you," I whispered.

He said, "You got dinner for me? At this hour?"

"Of course I got dinner for you—you have to eat. Don't I know you wouldn't stop and get your own dinner?"

"Thank you, baby," he said.

How could I not forgive that man if he made a mistake? How could he not forgive me? But you have to build up the trust and the love. It takes time. And to be really honest, in the bad times, you just pray your spiritual center holds to help you find your way home again. With dinner.

Listen: God knows I'm not an expert on finding a spiritual center in anyone else's life. I can only tell you what works for me.

I hope you find your own way to forgiving a wrong done to you. Please remember, we all try to aspire to something higher, and when we succeed, it's just such a glorious victory. It's the last step in making you ready to share your life with another. It's the first step to perfect peace in your heart.

Do We Have to Be Perfect to Find That Perfect Peace?

Oh, sure—that's how I got to be so spiritual, because I'm so perfect. Tell that to my girlfriends.

I know I'm not there yet. I have so many weaknesses that block the way to that kind of spiritual completeness. For example, I know God is still working on me getting out of my own way. For every blessing I have, for every gift I've been given, I tend to second-guess it. I don't stand comfortably in a space that God has created for me. I'll declare that I want and need a special something to be really happy, and then when it comes, I'll question it—do I deserve this? Is it right I should have it? Is this going to be what I ultimately want, or am I going to be disappointed in my choice? Should I wait for something better to come along?

That's a real flaw, this second-guessing of my blessings.

It's also very hard for me to focus on character, rather than reputation. I have to work hard not to be concerned with what others think of me. I have to be more focused on who I am and whether or not I am that person I proclaim to be. This huge character flaw in me—one which is the opposite of a spiritual approach to life—makes me far too needy for applause. It's hard when you're in show business not to care, but I can just hear God saying to me, "You don't need to work that hard for approval; I've already given you everything you need. It's yours. Stand in that space."

I keep trying.

God's Box: How Do You Pray?

For me, the all-controlling one, it's very hard to take my hands off the steering wheel. It's my nature to handle the details, all by myself. But think of it: if you ask God for help and then try to manipulate, deal, arrange everything yourself—why the heck are you asking God for help?

I figured out a way to stop myself. I started to envisage a box—a plain box, like a shoebox. In my mind, I called it the Something for God to Do box. When I desperately needed help or a blessing, I'd pray to God—then put the problem in God's box.

"This is now in the Something for God to Do box," I'd remind myself. "He's handling this one." Then, I'd step back.

Of course, you have to be willing to take the direction from God, when it comes—even if you don't like what you're hearing from above. I find that inevitably, God's box will empty out—problems solved.

✳ Still the voices in your head, and although you can pray anywhere, it's helpful to find a regular, quiet place; that becomes your sacred space, your altar, your reminder of God. Sit down. Talk. Listen.

✳ Try to cleanse your spirit of negativity, of angry thoughts, of revenge. Bring a joyful and sweet attitude to prayer.

✳ Don't ask God for specifics—ask for direction. Deepak Chopra once said that you best make things happen if you send out a prayer or an intention into the universe, take your hands off the steering wheel, and let the universe handle the details.

✳ Be open to a change in direction. Don't give out complicated vibes and messages; talk to your higher spirit sweetly, simply, and most of all, patiently. Can't rush God. I love the message I once read in the Koran, the Muslim bible: "O ye who believe! Seek help with patient persever-ance and prayer; for God is with those who patiently persevere."

✳ Try to believe in a higher spirit and pray with courage and love. But here's a miracle: even if you don't believe, it'll work. Studies have shown that critically ill patients got better much faster when people prayed for them than if they had no people praying for them. And lis-ten to this—*it didn't matter that the patients weren't believers.* What does that tell you, Kendra?

✳ Deepak again: "Surrender," he says in *The Book of Secrets.* "Give full at-tention, give appreciation of life's riches, open yourself to what is in front of you, don't be judgmental, be receptive to all possibilities, allow love to enter your life, and let God show up if He wants to. Again—pay attention: nothing is random, your life is full of signs and symbols."

    Maybe God is sending you one.

✳ Spiritual growth is spontaneous. Don't make plans. There's an old saying: "If you want to make God laugh, tell him about your plans." God will make the plans, do the work, and help you open to the un-known *if* you have a receptive mind. That means listen to your intu-ition, your dreams, and recurring themes in books and conversations. I can't remember where I read it, but someone very smart once said, "Seek insights on a path to spirituality, but don't order insights on demand." Ageless wisdom is available if you let go of old, sour thoughts and make room for new visions.

❊ It's my feeling that to establish a relationship with God, we ought to speak in our own words, not use someone else's words. Divine communication is yours for the asking, so ask in your own voice.

❊ Perhaps we ought to stop looking at God as if he were one of those pop-up Pez candy dispensers—in his case, a blessing dispenser. Don't worry, he's paying attention—and he calls 'em as he sees 'em.

❊ Wake up from a spiritual anesthesia. Program your mind for clarity, for being aware, for living in the moment. Take inspirations from the whole world, whether you're Christian, Jewish, Muslim, Buddhist, Hindu.

Talking to God and Tolerance for Others' Spiritual Conversations

All of the above is how I see it, anyway. In these difficult and terrifying days of nations warring as they invoke the name of God, of people who claim God to be their very own castigating others who also claim God as their own, I had some serious questions:

How can one prepare herself spiritually to be all she can be, if she's still secretly wondering whether her own religion is the best or only way to connect to God—no matter what her parents tell her? And even more troubling, how can anyone be sure that her god hears her? Is there something we all should know about praying so we can be sure God is listening?

It seemed appropriate to ask the experts. I chose three prominent leaders within three major religious groups. Here is how they see spirituality.

Question: How Can You Be Faithful to Your Own
Religion and Still Have Respect for Others?

Pastor A. R. Bernard, my own spiritual adviser, founder
and leader of the Christian Cultural Center in Brooklyn,
New York, a congregation of about 27,000 worshippers

Here's a reality: when we talk about Christianity, we're not just talking about a religion; we're talking about what Christians absolutely believe to be the truth. And the nature of truth is that it is exclusive, it's absolute. The moment we Christians accept the Biblical record and the truth of what Jesus said about himself, that truth becomes exclusive—because everything can't be true. There's something else: the moment we declare a truth, we also declare that everything else is false. Jesus said about himself, "I am the truth." He didn't say he was one of many truths, he said he was *the* truth. That is the Christian faith.

Now, this idea is attacked by many other religions that come from a more pluralistic view that embraces other faiths as alternate paths to God. In doing so, these faiths reject the notion that there's one path and one path alone, but in that rejection, they themselves become exclusive because they exclude the concept of only one path to God.

Thus, as a matter of fact, every religion is exclusive, because when you come down to it, there are always basic tenets of faith which the believer insists is *the* path, *the* way. Even if I were to take the Universalist's view of religion, which says all paths lead to God, again I'd be exclusive because I'd be saying Universalism is the only right way to believe.

Every religion, including Christianity, is exclusive.

So, how can Christianity, an exclusive religion, peacefully coexist in a world in which many faiths exist? How can I as a Christian who knows that Christ is the only truth, accept your path?

Well, of course I can't accept your path. But I can accept your choice. We can live together in this world because we do not judge. Jesus said, "Whosoever wills to come to him as the light, let him come." He has given us a marvelous gift called positive freedom—the power of choice. It's as if Jesus says, I offer you a path, you have the power to choose that path or make your own. If you choose to make your own path, I cannot promise you the path to Heaven—but that is always your choice.

So, how do you stay faithful to your own faith, never waver from believing your way is the only right way—and still live in peace with others? By accepting other people's choices for themselves. God respects that. He does not force himself on anyone. And I, as a Christian, will never deny the exclusiveness of my own truth, but I must respect, even if I don't accept, the truths of others: I respectfully allow choice to others, just as Christ does.

Rabbi Peter J. Rubinstein, senior rabbi of Central Synagogue, New York City

One should be able to believe in the possibility of conflicting truths. The Hebrew word for God is in the plural. I believe that Jews were signaled that our claim on a particular approach to God did not mean that other people didn't have the right to claim God in different ways. The reason why the Talmud is so many volumes is because it never provides only one accepted position: it gives conclusions, and then leaves it to us to assess the discussions that helped the scholars reach the conclusions. The Talmud cites the authoritative opinion and the differing views of others. These are counterpoints and *no one* is denigrated. I think the Talmud gives honor to all opinions across the spectrum because it says—sometimes *THIS* is so, and sometimes *THAT* is so. Only God ultimately knows the truth. We, with our individual ideas of God, may think we approach the truth, but the nature of being human and not divine is that we will never know whether what we believe is *the* single truth.

It would be the worst hubris to believe that only we know what God says. Others' ways of thinking and believing constantly challenge me to refine my own. I would like to know for certain how God wishes us to live and behave, but the only thing I know for sure is that I don't know anything for sure.

I do believe that the history of the Jewish people has given rise to a great sensitivity about God's ways and the way we're supposed to treat other people: that is why we *must* accept conflicting truths. To me, it is of vital importance to have multi-faith conversations in our world. Every person should have sufficient humility to say, "I have room in my life for those who speak differently about God, and who allow me to do the same."

Sheikh Abdullah Adhami, outstanding Muslim scholar of the noble lineage of the family of the prophet Muhammad, and a leader in the North American Islamic community

How can we be faithful to our own religion and still have respect for others' faiths? This is a central and perennial concern. From our Islamic perspective, every person is *born* faithful, born loving her creator, born yearning to be closer to her creator. People yearn for the freedom to worship God. It is a primordial spiritual essence within all of us that we are brought home to with an irresistible force—and that we can neither deny nor run away from. Along the journey of life, we encounter various obstacles and trials in our path of faithfulness. Aside from our own feebleness, one of the biggest obstacles we face is the people whose dogma and extremism actually lead us away from what faithfulness is supposed to be. Ironically, to the extremists—of every religion—people who have been scared away from "religion" appear to be disconnected, godless, and secular. These are the innumerable church, mosque, and synagogue refugees who are the products of self-righteousness and excess.

From a true Islamic perspective, there is one religion, one path, one God, one law, one system. God did not change his mind when he sent Moses, then sent Jesus, then Muhammad. Moses represents the Majesty of God *(jalâl)*. Jesus represents the forgiveness and beauty of God *(jamâl)*. Muhammad represents the sublime perfection of God *(kamâl)*. May God's peace be upon them all. I believe that if we had one universal religious language, there would be no disagreement about God, the one and only. True people of faith, true believers in God will have different but not conflicting ideas. Certainly, humans can be feeble and prone to error when they claim their own manifestation of a certain religious idea to be the only path to follow, but that's because of our human limitations. I categorically believe that true Muslims, Christians, Jews, Buddhists are all talking about the same thing—the sublime majesty and power of a universal God. That is why, in Islam, we can be faithful to our own religion and must always have respect for the faith of others.

Question: How Do You Pray to God?
How Do You Know if He Hears?

Pastor A. R. Bernard

First of all, to whom do we pray? As a Christian, I believe, as the geneticist Dean Hamer said in his book *The God Gene*, that we all have a genetic disposition to spirituality—a built-in desire to find ourselves in the divine. But, for me, the revelation of God in Christ holds that man is incapable of discovering the Divine by himself, even if we have a genetic inclination toward faith; thus it's necessary that the Divine reveal himself. And Christians believe that he did just that—in the person of Jesus Christ.

So, it's easy to pray to a divinity who is a person, and personal in the very body of Christ. Jesus understands human frailty, is sensitive to our condition because he was one of us. I believe that to pray to an animal, a statue, or a tree is to make no connection whatsoever with God: it's simply not the same as praying to another human being.

So, we pray, and all prayer is, is an invitation to communicate with God. But prayer must have two elements: one must pray in spirit and in truth. There has to be a connection between God and the very heart of you (not the facade you show the world). You must always, always pray in truth. And prayer is not about reciting something—we don't have to read from books as long as we communicate in heart and spirit.

If we can talk to God, believe that he can talk back to you. But how can we be sure that God hears us?

Trust the deep knowingness inside you, the sense of confidence and assurance you have while and after you pray. The sense of calm and knowingness is how you know God hears. Christians believe absolutely that the Divine Intelligence hears and speaks to us.

And where should one pray? Well, we don't go to church to be religious; we go to church to be spiritual. And we don't go to church to have a relationship with God, we go to church because of a relationship with God. So, this is important—prayer should not be confined only to a church, a mosque, or a synagogue. Jesus said, "Your body is the temple of Christ, so once you enter a relationship with

God, your body becomes a temple—and you carry that temple with you, everywhere you go." Thus, you can pray anywhere you go.

Do we have to be good to be spiritual? You are a good person as a result of entering a relationship with God. What's required for true spirituality is a belief in the revelation of God. We don't get to heaven based on our own bodies or work; we get to heaven solely on faith in the word of Christ.

Rabbi Peter J. Rubinstein

I think we have to make a distinction between worship and prayer. Worship involves community prayers, rites, and rituals. For the Jew, being part of the community is important. Worship doesn't need to take place in a sanctuary but needs the presence of the community. The Jew says, "my personal relationship with God is important but not only for me as an individual. God made a covenant with an entire people. If the world's going to get better, it will happen in the midst of community. My individual salvation can be accomplished in the salvation of the community on every level—my family community, my Jewish community, my city, my nation, my world."

I want to add that health is part of prayer. My body is God's gift and when my body feels well, chances are my soul will feel well. I believe you have to care for yourself so that you're able to take care of your family and then the larger community. Health becomes part of the totality of what humans are at their best. You must be the healthiest you can be but you need to know that even when struck by a nefarious disease, you still can be healthy in spirit and feel the rhythm of creation.

Personal prayer is different from worship. There are prayers of thanksgiving to acknowledge the gifts one has in life and there are prayers of blessing. When I bless my children in my home on *Shabbat* nights, I would love God to answer my prayers for them. But does God hear those petitional prayers of mine? I don't know. One cannot know whether God hears. But, the blessing does more than ask God to answer. The prayer itself provides strength for me, and for those who have been blessed.

I think that prayers of petition in which we ask God to do something for us alone, are presumptuous as we try to make deals with God, with the idea that God will automatically respond to our prayers if we're good enough. That is not my definition of prayer. For me, praying to the God in whom I believe is, in itself, a force that strengthens me, and that is a perfect response from God. If you have a certainty about how God behaves, then you believe you have power over God.

But I don't have such certainty and I don't believe a prayer should ask, "What's good for me?" I think that a prayer should not expect that God will cure and fix everything for me. In my relationship with God, I ask that God help me with the strength and the dignity to face whatever challenges, victories, or tragedies confront me. My act of praying does that. When I pray, it is for the purpose of losing myself in a conversation with God, to free myself of intellectualism and rationality, to believe that God will provide me with calm, comfort, and strength to do what I have to do. That's how I pray. That's what I pray. That's what I really need.

Sheikh Abdullah Adhami

God categorically hears our prayers. There is no doubt about that.

How should we pray? There are two forms of "prayer" in Islamic tradition. One is the realm of remembering and exaltation of the Divine through supplication, invocation, and benediction. This can be a continual process that requires only the presence of heart and mind. The other is the *salah,* from the Arabic "to connect." It is akin to the Aramaic *(shelayvah)* and Hebrew *(shalah)* for "to be at ease; to have quiet; [and also] to prosper." It is the distinctive physical act of kneeling and genuflection at prescribed times of the day. It is a cosmic "connection" with one's world. It involves the same physical limbs that one utilizes in the earthly, temporal world. These faculties are gifts that one is entrusted with, and how one chooses to use them can either honor or debase. The ritual washing preceding the Muslim prayer is a spiritual cleansing of one's limbs to prepare the mortal human to connect with the eternal, heavenly realm.

Women in particular are endowed with a spiritual preeminence that stems from their devotion to genuineness and belonging. It is a yearning for what is viscerally authentic in all their connections and relationships—especially with God. It is this very essence that makes woman profoundly soulful in her giving and at once so insatiable in her yearning. It is also what makes her so bewilderingly enigmatic, so disarmingly incomprehensible—even to herself. Ironically, it is also this gift that makes her appear tentative, often uncertain—when all that she wishes is for everything that she ever does to be meaningful, authentic, and pure. Women usually need privacy when they pray to replenish their formidable repertoire of giving, though their very essence is a form of prayer; their speech is prayer; and—as distinct from their whims—their feelings are prayer too. Devotion is the secret behind a woman's eloquence and the essence of her virtue. Incidentally, this is epitomized by Mary in the Quran, and Fatimah in the prophetic tradition.

In Islam, spirituality is inseparable from life. It's connected to personal morality, a sense of what's good and right, and what's wrong. Taken to its ultimate sensibility, this means that human failing, vileness, and error exist at every level in society. Religious leaders (priests, rabbis, and imams) are human—and are neither infallible nor exempt from accountability to those that they are privileged and entrusted with serving. The transgression or error of a member of the clergy does not—and should not—control your personal spirituality. Your true connection with God is a personal and moral responsibility—requiring no human intermediary. This bond helps us to acknowledge our spiritual essence and is stronger than everyone's human frailties. It is through reaching out to God that we heal and grow.

Prayer is language, and I really think that God created language to express to us how special we are. Conversely, prayer and language is a way to show God our devotion, our genuineness, and that is why we pray—each in her own way.

A Simple Prayer

My spiritual adviser, Pastor Bernard, says that Jesus was very aware that some of us simply didn't know how to pray. The Lord's Prayer is Jesus' response to those who asked, "How do we pray?"

"Pray like this," said Jesus.

The Lord's Prayer

Our Father, who art in heaven,
Hallowed be thy name.
Thy Kingdom come,
Thy will be done,
On Earth as it is in heaven.
Give us this day our daily bread
And forgive us our trespasses,
As we forgive those who trespass against us.
And lead us not into temptation,
But deliver us from evil.
For thine is the kingdom,
And the power,
And the glory,
Forever and ever.
Amen.

The Lord's Prayer is so simple, but it gives us all the ingredients that should go into prayer. I love it. Here are some ways to break the prayer down, according to some spiritual friends of mine:

Our Father in heaven: This teaches us to whom to address our prayers—the Father, the source of strength.

Hallowed be your name: This tells us to worship God and praise him simply as the Master of all.

Your kingdom come, your will be done: This reminds us that we're to pray for God's plan and God's will to prevail in our lives—not our own plan and desires.

Give us today our daily bread: We're encouraged to ask God for the basics we really need.

Forgive us our debts, as we have forgiven our debtors: This reminds us to turn from our sins and forgive others, as we've been forgiven by God.

Lead us not into temptation . . . deliver us from evil: Here's a plea for help in victory over sin, and a request for protection from the attacks of those who would harm us.

For yours is the kingdom, and the power, and the glory, forever and ever: Here's our acknowledgment that God is the source of all, and our fondest wish is to be with him in eternity.

If you're searching, this plain but powerful prayer should give you the comfort, joy, peace, and answers you seek.

Part Four

Doing It! Making Lifestyle Changes

Chapter 12

The Happy Route to Change:
Fail-Safe Ways to Rev Up Your Lifestyle

S hould you try to change?

Well, if you can think like a lawyer and you've won almost every "case" in your life; if you were pleased with the results of all your self-assessments; if you're totally right with the way you look, feel, and relate to the Man upstairs; if you're perfect (or even a shade less than perfect)—you don't have to do another thing to change your lifestyle.

Riiiight. Perfection happens a lot.

But if you have looked yourself clear in the eye and seen places where you might consciously change your health, relationships, emotional attitude, look, or spiritual well-being for the better, get a pencil and notebook.

Because, the next question is—specifically, *how* do you do change? Are there exercises you can employ to help yourself become stronger, physically and spiritually?

There sure are. The following are fine ways to become the best you can be and truly get ready to meet love and romance around the next corner. If you've gotten this far in this book, you've changed your life already: you now know how to assess yourself, look deeply inward, and figure out places you can change for the best.

Here's the route:

Make a decision to change one thing—only one at a time—either the way you dress or shop, the way you deal with your spiritual self, your exercise regimen, the way you deal with a relationship in your life. Write down your intention (declarations seem to last better when they're in black and white). Give yourself a time span in which to accomplish your goal. For example, you might say, "By June, I will have toned my body, lost twenty pounds, found my best makeup, found a way to speak with God, and met the man of my dreams."

Probably not going to happen. You've got to make your intention realistic. By June, for example, there ain't no way you'll find the perfect lipstick. Chill out with the unattainable.

Keep your declaration to one or two sentences. If you need a page to state your intention, it's too complicated to work. I'd already lost about fifty pounds when I met Al, but when we started talking about getting married, I realized one day that I still weighed more than he did. Your Star did not love that insight. About four months before our wedding, I decided I wanted to weigh less than my husband on our wedding day. That didn't seem too much to ask.

In the past, I'd always focused on the way I felt to tell me how much weight I needed to lose, but just this once, I made a decision to change by the numbers. I wrote a note to myself saying that on the day of my wedding, I would weigh a certain amount of pounds, quite a bit less than what I'd weighed for years.

And I did.

Since the wedding, incidentally, I've never again focused on numbers. I'm still losing weight, but now I focus on being able to run up a flight of stairs or walk the neighborhood with Al—without getting out of breath. And I do.

Follow through with action. Take the Nike approach—Just do it. When you're satisfied that you've made a change for the better that will *probably* last, tackle another area. Keep track of your progress in the journal. Date each entry.

Bring in a second or third party, a trusted witness to your action. Sometimes, making a life change is easier if you do it with someone else: you can monitor each other's victories and commiserate with each other each time you fall back. Sometimes, even just declaring your intentions to a trusted third party helps you stay steadfast to your goal.

Reevaluate yourself in three months. Are you holding fast to your intention? Great! But if not, don't throw in the towel. Go back to number 1, and start again. You get as many turns as you need. You'll need them, momma. If you make just one major life change (exercise more, break a bad relationship or start a good one, learn to achieve a monied look without spending a fortune, find peace in spirituality)—even just one lifestyle change—it's well worth the price of this book, right?

Fail-safe Ways to Rev Up Your Lifestyle

Sometimes, in addition to changing things about your body, your psyche, and your spiritual awareness, you simply want to make life more interesting, more textured. There's no question that a person who feels secure and blessed, who has many layers to her personality will attract more like-minded people. Revving up your lifestyle makes you more ready to meet and recognize the love of your life.

None of the following requires a huge commitment, and all are guaranteed to make you feel more whole, more energetic, more appealing, more knowing. Try one, try them all: eventually, I promise you, your best self will emerge.

1. Take a Calculated Risk

I'm sure there are 200 million women out there as I write this who are kicking themselves because they missed chances—and they missed them because of fear of the unknown. We tend to think to ourselves: I'll look like a jerk; I'm not good at this; I'm making a fool of myself. I think too many of us take too few risks because we tend to misread the word *risk*. We see handling our own investment portfolios, initiating a connection with a new guy, taking a course in improvisational acting, moving to another city, or severing a toxic friendship as a do-or-die situation—if we risk and we fail, we're dead. Failure means it's all over. Failure's kind of shameful. And so, many smart women traditionally re-move themselves from the art of taking risks. It's a pity.

Here's what I think: failure does not mean it's all over. Failure's not at all shameful. There's nothing like taking a risk to make you feel daring, excited, aware, and privy to the infinite possibilities of life—even if you fail. There's one caveat: instead of taking plain old zany risks, we should take calculated risks. What the difference? A zany risk is a rash gamble—based just on chance—kind of Las Vegas style. A calculated risk means using available information to esti-mate whether you'll succeed or fail. A zany risk is going out alone with a cute guy you met on the subway. It's a rash gamble because he may be a cute ax murderer, for all you know. A calculated risk is asking your friend to set you up with her boyfriend's brother. Available information: you know your friend's boyfriend, you know how he was raised, you like his style—chances are, you're going to like his brother. And he probably isn't an ax murderer or you would have heard. Driving to work on a busy highway, flying in a jet plane, or investing in a new but well-researched stock are risks, but because you know the statistics of crashing or losing all your money are low, they're calculated risks, in other words—low risk. Taking a social risk—initiating a conversation with a fascinating stranger at a party or signing up for a salsa class—is a low, calculated risk. Skydiving and playing the wheel of fortune are not calculated risks. When you take a calculated risk where the odds are more on your side than against, you have a good chance to gain joy or maybe big bucks, and you feel terrific. You've made your life more interesting. If you've lost, you haven't lost everything, you haven't failed; in-stead, you're getting in the habit of taking reasonable chances and opening yourself up for success. Eleanor Roosevelt once said, "You must do the thing you think you cannot do."

It was a calculated risk for me to begin my journey to make myself physically, emotionally, and spiritually more ready for love. I could have failed, but chances are, I wouldn't have. I thought I'd gone as far as I could, but in reality, I was out on a limb—and I'd stopped short right there at the end. I had to take a chance and go beyond the limb, I had to jump and find my parachutes along the way. If I hadn't gotten all that stuff together before I stepped off that limb though, my journey to finding love would have been a dumb risk. I wasn't com-plete—how could I expect to find Al? I had to prepare for the jump and then I'd have backup, a built-in parachute: it would be a more perfect, able, and confident me.

A last thing about risk taking. Temper it with your trusted intuition. Sometimes, no matter what the evidence says, there's a "knowing" in your gut that will tell you something different. Respect your intuition. See number 2 below.

2. Trust Your Intuition

Intuition is not hot emotion. It is not a hope or fear. It usually arrives with calmness. If you feel passionately and strongly about something, wait a few moments for your emotions to cool down; then, you can more clearly hear your intuition. What will you hear? Intuition has been defined in many ways, but I like best the sense of quiet knowing. It's also been referred to as a strong hunch or a gut feeling. Others call it getting vibes about certain decisions you have to make or people whom you meet. Figure it this way: if your senses extended further than you've thought possible, if you were connected to more things than you knew existed—that's intuition working. It works all the time without your even realizing it, and it brings vital information to your attention without your asking for it. No one quite understands how intuition comes about, but I believe it's real and that it functions on physical, emotional, and spiritual levels. Sometimes, you just know when a person you've recently met will be terrific for you (that's how I felt about Al). Sometimes you just know a person will be more destructive than instructive. Whether you're responding to old or new friends or making a decision that might jump-start a new business or lifestyle for yourself, allow intuition to play a part.

Here's a caveat: when you feel a strong hunch or an intuitive vibe, it's a great idea to test it with some logic and reasoning before acting on it. Ask questions of yourself: is this insane, is it impossible, or is there a good reason why I might feel this strong hunch? A fine balance of thought, logic, and intuition is what you're reaching for.

Everyone possesses intuition, but some people are more highly developed intuitively than others. Can you strengthen your intuition? Yes. I did it. Before I started getting ready for love, my intuition in directing my own career was flawless. My intuition with relationships with women friends and colleagues—flawless. But my relationships with the men in my life were deeply flawed. I found myself giving, giving, giving to men who were not worthy of my time and who didn't respond in the same ways I gave. I was trying to fit square-peg men into round holes without realizing how square they were. I had to learn to trust the little voice inside that said, No square-peg men, Star—you deserve to be with someone who thinks you're the most wonderful person on the planet. Funny thing: when you've become the best you can be, you *do* deserve him.

Many say that paying close attention to the way your whole body responds to people, information, and situations helps develop intuition. Do you tense up, perhaps perspire, perhaps tighten your facial muscles at certain encounters or suggestions others give you? Your intuition is saying, beware. But sometimes, does your whole body react in a joyful but tuned-in and aware posture that says, trust your gut? Then, trust it.

What if you always distrust your intuition and are skeptical it even exists? Keep an open mind, girl. Scientists have shown that we use only about a tenth of our thinking abilities, and intuition may well figure into that vast, unused capability to help you make the best decisions for yourself.

3. Practice Mindfulness

Thich Nhat Han is a Vietnamese Buddhist monk who has popularized the extraordinary and freeing concept of mindfulness. In its simplest form, it means paying attention to the simplest details of life. If you have to wash the pots after dinner, and you hate washing pots, try this: as you wash, pay attention to the way the warm water looks and feels as it splashes your hands. Carefully focus in on the silver of the pot, the way the sponge makes it gleam, the sense of satisfaction you have as each food lump is scraped away. Watch the soap slide down the drain to—where?

Paying exquisite attention like this makes the mind go completely still, and gives a sense of pleasure and fulfillment instead of anger. Practice mindfulness the next time you're caught in a traffic jam. Concentrate on the way each car slowly stops, focus in on the way the motion of the car soothes and quiets. Feel how the sun warms your arm as it rests on the car window frame. Feel the vibration of the motor. Immerse yourself in the experience until your frustration at being in that traffic jam flies out the window.

When you eat, practice mindfulness—it's a lifestyle change that can lead to an appreciation of the texture of the food you're eating, the smell, the color, the juices that explode in your mouth. Be conscious of the way each bite feels in your mouth, pay attention to your mouth as you chew. Eat slowly. Focus in. You'll find that you're eating with far more appreciation and not gorging on food out of habit. Mindfulness. It changes your life, minute by minute.

4. Choose Your Friends: Don't Settle for Being Chosen

My mom always used to tell me that "people know you by whom you affiliate with." As usual, Momma was right. Why settle for a needy person saying, "You're cool, I want to hang with you"? Instead, it's so much more fulfilling for you to say to an interesting or very good person, "You're cool—let's hang for a while."

Friendships are like all relationships. Everyone should bring something to the table. If you find you're the only one bringing, don't feel guilty about cutting the friendship. For me, that means I hope you will be bringing an emotional connection, a spiritual connection, or even just making me laugh to our friendship table, so at the end of our time together, I should be better off for spending it with you. Of course, that goes both ways: I also am very aware that I must bring something to that table, and I'll work my butt off to do that—you better believe it.

Absolute

True friends don't mind carrying you as long as there's finally a destination to which you can carry yourself.

There is nothing more conducive to a lifestyle change than bringing a new, loving, vital friend into your life—or on the other hand, ridding yourself of a toxic, destructive friend even though you've known her forever and it makes you feel guilty to cut an old-time bond. But cut it you must: a friend who is toxic will eventually hurt you.

Who's a toxic friend? I try not to have in my life any friend who

* never brings new ideas, laughs or loyalty to the table.
* seems to try to control me (control often looks like helping—be careful).
* wants to be my friend only for what I can do for her. This friend is a user—and thus, a loser in my book.
* has betrayed me. When someone betrays you by gossiping, telling your secrets, or breaking a promise, it hurts deeply. That's taking away from the table, not bringing to it.
* is all me, me, me, me—and enough about me, what do you think of me? Self-centered people bring only their own egos to the table. That's not enough to be my friend forever.
* uses me as a leaning post. Often, very needy people choose famous, rich, or powerful people to be their friends. I may choose to help you sometimes—but real friendship with a too-needy person? Not possible.
* is a one-upper. One-uppers are people who always have to jump one step ahead of me. I love my friends to challenge me, but when I sense that someone is being ultracompetitive to squash me, I steer clear. That's not a true friend.
* is a judge, not an advocate. Judgmental people who seem to criticize and find fault with all my decisions are not terrific for my confidence. I try to be a friend who sticks up for and supports my girls—not tears down their egos.

5. Give Back

There's a Bible directive that I believe in with all my heart and I've written a little about this on page 218.

"Much is required from those to whom much has been given" (Luke 12:48). I look around, and I thank God for all that has been given me, and then, I give back. It's not because I'm good or sweet or kind—it's because the Bible tells me I must. It's a directive.

You there—reading these words, please look around. Is there good health in your life, are there friends of your heart, can you put a meal on your table without asking anyone for help, can you rely on your own intelligence, do you own courage? If you can say yes to any one of these, let alone all, much has been given. Give back. It may be the very best way to prepare yourself for finding the biggest love in your life.

I started with my own family, who have been my rock, my inspiration from the beginning. Because so much has been given to me from them, do you know what joy it gave me to buy my parents a home, write a check for the whole thing—no mortgage payments, no taxes for them? Do you know how good I feel that I can pay for a companion to come in several hours a week to hang with my grandfather, to play checkers with him, to help him walk around the neighborhood so he can still get fresh air? And my grandmother—who has been a bigger ally? Now a lady can come in to help my grandmother with her home so she has a moment to take a shower, watch a soap opera or her granddaughter on *The View.*

I could pay back every dime of the $70,000 I received in school loans. And because of my public life and even because of the pain-in-the-butt media, I could go further than my own family and debts and bring any public appeal I have to highlight community organizations like God's Love We Deliver, Dress for Success, and Girls Incorporated, where I can mentor young women.

The glorious Oprah helped me here. She once said, "Star, at one point you'll have to realize you're special. They always say that everyone is created equal and everyone has the opportunity to do the same things, but in some ways that's not true. That's because some of us have really been given more than others. When you embrace the fact that God has given you so much, stand in that space, accept it, and understand the responsibility."

I buy that totally. There's a responsibility to give back that goes along with fame and accolades but there's also a responsibility to give back if you have ever felt lucky about anything in your life.

Give back. In a million different ways, it changes your life and the way you feel about yourself. You've acquitted your responsibility. Good girl.

6. Meditate

There have been too many positive studies on meditation for the following to be wrong: if you can quiet your mind for only about fifteen minutes a day, your brain will work differently and better. Angst won't feel as—well, anxious. Scientists have told us that mind-calming hormones are actually released when one meditates or prays (and the latter is how I personally meditate). There's no mystery in meditation: it works even before you know it's working. The trick is to learn how to give your attention to one thing without thinking about anything else. Stress flies out the window—sometimes for a short time, but sometimes for a very long time.

Here's one way to meditate: Sit or stand silently in a quiet place and close your eyes. If you choose to sit, place your hands palm up on your thighs. If you're standing, let your arms hang loosely by your sides. Let go, lose it, will your stress to be out of there. Repeat one single word or a phrase over and over and over. If that bores you too much, concentrate on the way your belly moves in and out as you breathe. Or the way your tongue hangs loose in your mouth. Or speak to God.

Prayerful meditation sweeps the clutter of uneasy thoughts from your mind. Calmness prevails. Feel tranquility. Feel bliss.

7. Find an Intercessor

My friend Elena is my prayer partner and my intercessor with God. Everyone should have a trusted person who interposes on her behalf when praying—it's like an insurance policy, it's double prayer. Whenever anything is going on in my life, negative or positive, she prays for me. For example, I'll say to Elena, "I'm about to make a decision [she doesn't even have to know the subject of my decision]—please keep me in your prayers."

I know what her prayer will consist of: "Dear God," she'll say, "please direct Star to make a decision that will be to your glory."

I am Al's intercessor. I pray for him constantly without him knowing it or knowing that he needs it. Al's mother is also Al's prayer intercessor. And if you think prayer doesn't work, if you've never been religious or spiritual, just go back to that moment when you desperately needed help or advice, when you were terrified and just didn't know what to do, and you prayed anyway—and everything calmed down.

It's a blessing to have someone who prays for you.

8. Celebrate Yourself

It's not conceited and it's not selfish to love yourself. How in the world can anyone else love you if you don't think you're worth it? In fact, if you live with self-respect and self-love, you don't need the world to tell you how great you are, you don't need the constant stroking that some people require. It's the people who do not celebrate themselves or recognize their own value who need to seize all the attention because of their insecurity. These people don't even believe it when others tell them they're terrific because deep inside, they obsess on their own weaknesses. If you constantly find fault with yourself, I'll bet that you look for the worst in others, as well.

So, bask in the glory of who you are and whom you will become. Be friendly to you—never limit your options. Choose to disagree with those who want to put you down (of course, always check inside to see if there is any truth to what the bad-talking person bad-talks.)

Here's a truism: don't let 'em dog you out. When someone dogs you out, it strikes a blow to your self-esteem. Don't let anyone else say what you're about or put you in a box. You know, my motto is "I am the author of the only dictionary that defines me." If you've worked hard at being the best you can be, if you know yourself as a good person, you can define yourself that way and freely celebrate yourself. People who love you know who you are. Everybody else, doesn't.

9. Finally—the Premarital Solution

This one is *sooooo* important. Trust your Auntie Star.

Say you've prepared spiritually, emotionally, and physically, and you've found each other! Well, congratulations—but there's still a little more work to be done. This is actually the most interesting part.

Premarital counseling is an idea whose time has come. America has the world's highest divorce rate—half of all marriages fail. Incredible! The irony of this is that most people spend far more time planning their wedding than preparing for their marriage. The first time most couples will ever see a marriage counselor or any expert in the subleties of what will be the most important relationship in their lives is when they're in despair and trying to avoid a divorce, when they're trying to find things in their ruined marriage to salvage.

Doesn't it make sense to spend a little time *before* the marriage ceremony finding out how to discuss differences in ways that actually strengthen a relationship and make intimacy—well, more intimate? You bet it does, Kendra.

Here's a statistic: the number one predictor of divorce is the constant *avoidance* of conflict. Couples who don't know how to handle conflict eventually just shut down. Successful couples learn to dance in spite of their clumsiness and different styles.

These premarital courses are fascinating and offered all over the place. They include small group role-playing and lectures on strengths and weaknesses of individual couples, the incredibly complicated adventures you'll face as a couple in new parenting, sexual dysfunction issues that may arise, substance abuse, spousal abuse, depression issues, anger and communication issues, dual careers, and illness during a marriage. Some are secular courses connected to no religious base at all, and they're taught in community centers, in private offices, on military bases, and even at county courthouses across the country. Others are courses adapted for different religious denominations, and they're taught in churches, synagogues, and mosques. It's a good idea to take a course provided by a qualified expert, and these include psychiatrists and psychologists, clinical social workers, licensed marriage and family therapists, licensed mental health counselors, or an official representative of a religious organization who has had relevant training.

Let me say this: Al and I would never, ever in a million years have had a chance at a successful marriage had not Pastor Bernard suggested a premarital marriage course.

We were asked, for example, how we saw marriage during one of our counseling sessions. The following is how we each answered:

✳ Al
  - Covenant between two individuals and God
  - Incorporation of two lives and creation of one corporation
  - Bigger than the two of us . . . a calling to reproduce, teach, and spread the word of God
✳ Star
  - Lifetime commitment of love
  - Setting of common goals based on common desires
  - A union that is blessed and directed by God

And here are some marital absolutes we learned in premarital counseling.

Marital Absolutes

❧

Marriage is a confluence that flows,
rather than a collision that crashes.

Two people who live together are seeking involvement.
When two people get married, they are seeking commitment.

A wife is like a mirror in which a man sees himself.

continued

A woman finds security in a man's consistency.

A woman wants a man to be decisive, strong, and consistent.

A woman determines a man's strength by his gentleness.

A man's kindness is what makes him attractive to a woman.

Where are premarital courses given?

* You can find out about a religiously based premarital course from your religious leader.
* A good Web site to find out about secular premarital courses is http://www.smartmarriages.com.
* Your local marriage license bureau can also give you information about where local courses are offered.

Epilogue

There you have it: how to get ready physically, emotionally, and spiritually for the greatest relationship in your life.

Can you do it?

Ten years ago, I was sure I was ready for love. I wasn't. I didn't deserve to meet the Prince because I wasn't yet the best I could be. I wasn't bringing much to the table. It wasn't that I had nothing to bring—I had so much already. But I had stopped moving and was simply standing in place.

I needed to become a woman who was ready for change, who was open to possibility. I had to fix *me* in subtle and not so subtle ways—needed to rev up my assets, shed some skin, and rejuvenate. I had to first develop the greatest relationship not with a man but with a woman I was proud of—and that woman was Star. Once *I* was ready, in many important ways it wouldn't matter terribly if I never found *him*. I'd made myself the woman I wanted to be, so even if I ended up not meeting the man of my dreams right away, I was still in a win-win situation. I'd found the best *me*.

Today, when I walk out of a room and my husband says to me, "Let 'em have it, Ms. Jones, let 'em have it," it sends me over the moon. I found the best me, and then Al found me. I was ready for him.

If you've read this book, you will be ready soon. I know it. I feel you fulfilling your potential. I feel you growing. You can be so fine if you just put your mind to it. You will *shine.*

Luck and love to you, sister. I'm rooting for you, all the way. Feel it?

Acknowledgments

Giving honor to God with whom all things are possible. . . .

This is my time to acknowledge, thank and praise the people who helped make *Shine,* shine!

Sherry Suib Cohen, my writer, guru, confidant, friend and everyday example of love and devotion in marriage. Your ability to get in my head, organize my thoughts, and give life to my words is the sparkle in *Shine.*

Kathryn Huck, my editor (this book is your baby as much as mine . . .) and the rest of my Collins family, especially big boss Joe, Paul, and Jean Marie.

The Resources: Pastor A. R. Bernard (the most theologically anointed man I've ever met . . . I've learned more from you than anyone in my life; Grace and Peace my friend), Sheikh Abdullah Adhami (As-Salaam Alaikum), Rabbi Peter J. Rubinstein (Shalom), Sybil Evans, (led me to Sheikh Abdullah Adhami), Sister Malaak Shabazz (Malcolm X's daughter and a student of Islam), Sister Aisha H. L. al-Adawiya (curator at the Schomburg Center for Research in Black Culture), Ros Harber (liaison to Rabbi Rubinstein), Vincent Roppatte, Director of Beauty for Elizabeth Arden Salons/Saks Fifth Avenue, Mount Sinai Hospital's nutritionist, Rebecca Blake, Julie Aldefar and Fran Taylor, the women who keep me styled and sharp looking, beauty expert Paula Begoun and all the beauty consultants, personal shoppers, and sales associates who clue me in on the steals and deals before everyone else.

The Team: Mel Berger, my Literary Agent who brokered the deal, Lisa Davis, Esq., my lawyer who keeps it all legal, Elizabeth Meyer, my personal assistant who really belongs in that inner circle of my life because she has earned it, Shannon Walker, my assistant at *The View* who coordinates my life, Margarita Lozada, Al's assistant who coordinates his life and thus makes mine easier, my interns Ruthie and Laurie (thank you for formatting the manuscript), photographers, Charles and Jennifer Maring, Melanie Votaw who transcribed all the tapes of every interview, Brad Zeifman, and Karl Nilsson, my publicists and unofficial hand holders and firefighters;

. . . and Al Scales Reynolds for writing, editing, supporting, encouraging, and convincing me that being vulnerable in print is not a sign of weakness . . . but instead a sign of strength.

My parents, sister, family, and best friends, who are in that inner circle and protect me even when I don't know I need it . . .

and finally, the doctors (you know who you are), nutritionists, physical therapists, trainers, and supportive friends who saved my life and put me on the path to *shine* for the rest of my life.

Index